Veterinary Physiology
At A Glance

Veterinary Physiology At A Glance

By

Dr. Ashish Mishra
Senior Scientist
Animal Physiology Division
National Institute of Animal Nutrition and Physiology
Adugodi-560030
Bangluru, Karnataka, India

SSPH

SATISH SERIAL PUBLISHING HOUSE
403, Express Tower, Commercial Complex, Azadpur, Delhi-110033 (India)
Phone : 011-27672852, Fax : 91-11-27672046
E-mail : info@satishserial.com, hkjain1975@yahoo.com
Website : www.satishserial.com

Published by :

SATISH SERIAL PUBLISHING HOUSE

403, Express Tower, Commercial Complex, Azadpur, Delhi-110033 (INDIA)
Phone : 011-27672852 Fax : 91-11-27672046
E-mail : info@satishserial.com, hkjain1975@yahoo.com

ISBN 978-93-81226-98-8

Typeset at: Harminder Kharb *for* Laxmi Art Creation # 9971212252
Printed at: Salasar Imaging Systems, Delhi-110035

PREFACE

I feel happy to bring out this book entitled **"Veterinary Physiology At A Glance"** which will be helpful to all Veterinary graduate and post graduate students of all universities where Veterinary Physiology or Animal Physiology is being taught. This book is an outcome of compilation of objective questions and short notes on all the chapters of Veterinary Physiology syllabus from different sources presented in a simple, lucid and understandable language.

Veterinary Physiology is always interesting because it helps to understand the animal body system. Though numbers of Veterinary Physiology books are available nationally and internationally but here a sincere effort has been made to provide students an overall idea on this subject within a short period. Realizing the importance of Veterinary Physiology discipline in under graduate and post graduate courses there is need and demand of well illustrated explained questionaries in the form of book. To meet these requirements this book has been compiled. A sincere attempt has also been made to fulfil the requirements of present curriculum of Veterinary Physiology.

Progressive and constructive suggestions for improvement of this manuscript are welcome and appreciated.

(Ashish Mishra)

CONTENTS

CHAPTER-1

Cell

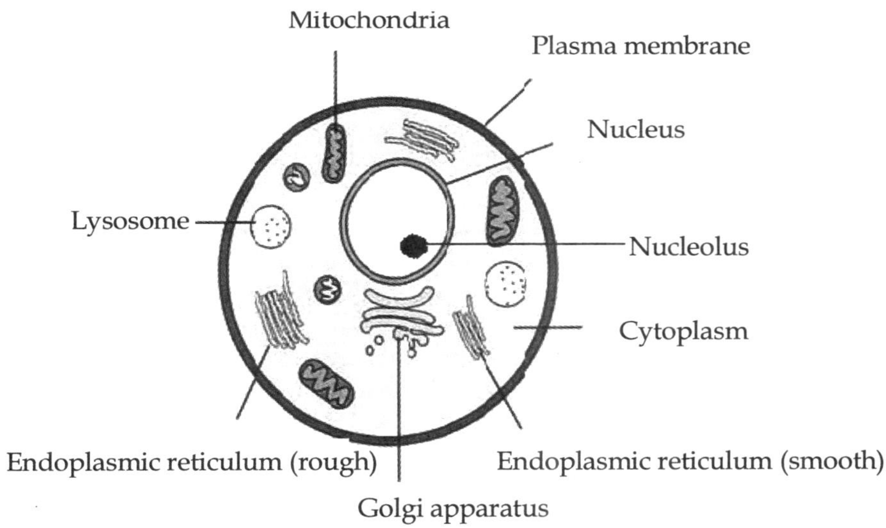

The cell is the basic and smallest units of life. There are millions of different types of cells. There are cells that are organisms onto themselves, such as microscopic amoeba and bacteria cells. There are also cells that only function as a part of a larger organism, such as the cells that make up total body. In the body, there are brain cells, skin cells, liver cells, stomach cells etc. All of these cells have unique functions and features. All cells have a skin called the **plasma membrane** or cell membrane, protecting it from the outside environment. The cell membrane regulates the movement of water, nutrients and wastes into and out of the cell. Inside of the cell membrane are the working parts of the cell. At the center of the cell there is

nucleus. The cell nucleus contains the cell's DNA, the genetic code that coordinates protein synthesis. In addition to the nucleus, there are many **organelles** inside of the cell that help to carry out the day-to-day operations of the cell. One important cellular organelle is the **ribosome**. Ribosomes participate in protein synthesis. The transcription phase of protein synthesis takes places in the cell nucleus. After this step the mRNA leaves the nucleus and travels to the cell's ribosomes, where translation occurs. Another important cellular organelle is the **mitochondria**. Mitochondria are often referred to as the power house of the cell because many of the reactions that equire energy take place in mitochondria. **Lysosomes** are organelles that contain enzymes that aid in the digestion of nutrient molecules and other materials.

There are two basic types of cells, primitive prokaryotes and the more complex eukaryotes. The cell structure of prokaryotes differs greatly from that of eukaryotes. Eukaryotes have "true" nuclei containing their DNA, whereas the genetic material in prokaryotes is not membrane-bound. Eukaryotic organisms may be unicellular as in amoeba or multicellular as in plants and animals. The defining characteristic in prokaryotes is the absence of a nucleus. The size of ribosomes in prokaryotes are smaller than in eukaryotes. The genomes of prokaryotes are held within an irregular DNA/protein complex in the cytosol called the **nucleoid**, which lacks a nuclear envelope. Prokaryotes generally lack membrane-bound cell compartments: such as mitochondria and chloroplasts. Both eukaryotes and prokaryotes contain large RNA/protein structures called ribosomes, which produce protein. Prokaryotes are usually much smaller than eukaryotic cells. Prokaryotes also differ from eukaryotes in that they contain only a single loop of stable chromosomal DNA stored in an area named the nucleoid, while eukaryote DNA is found on tightly bound and organized chromosomes. Prokaryotes and eukaryotes have some common characteristics as both the cells have DNA as their genetic material. Both the cells are covered by a cell membrane and contain RNA. Both the cells are made from the same basic chemicals like carbohydrates, proteins, nucleic acid, minerals, fats and vitamins. Both have similar basic metabolism processes like photosynthesis and reproduction which require a supply of energy and regulate the flow of the nutrients and wastes that enter and leave them. The organelles in eukaryotic cells allow them to perform more complex functions than prokaryotic cells.

The difference between plant cells and animal cells are that, animal cells are typical eukaryotic cell, enclosed by a **plasma membrane** and contain a membrane-bound nucleus and organelles. Unlike the cells of the two other eukaryotic kingdoms, plants and fungi, animal cells don't have a cell wall. Many animals have skeletons to give their body structure and support. Plants do not have a skeleton for support but have unique cellular structure called the **cell wall**. The cell wall is a rigid structure outside of the cell membrane composed mainly of the polysaccharide cellulose. In addition to the cell wall; plant cells contain an organelle called the **chloroplast**. Chloroplast allow plants to harvest energy from sunlight through pigments called chlorophyll.

Organelles in eukaryotic cells and their functions

i. Plasma membrane/Cell membrane

All living cells have a plasma membrane that encloses their contents. In prokaryotes, the membrane is the inner layer of protection surrounded by a rigid cell wall. Eukaryotic animal cells have only the membrane to contain and protect their contents. This membrane is a biological membrane that separates the interior of all cells from the outside environment. The cell membrane is selectively permeable to ions and organic molecules and controls the movement of substances in and out of cells. The plasma membrane is composed of two molecules as fats (phospholipids) and proteins. The fat is a phospholipid bilayer embedded with proteins. Some of the protein molecules form tiny channels in the membrane while others help transport substances from one side of the membrane to the other. Plasma membrane is involved in variety of cellular processes such as cell adhesion, ion conductivity and cell signaling. It also serves as the attachment surface for the extracellular glycocalyx and cell wall and intracellular cytoskeleton.

ii. Cytoplasm

Within the plasma membrane there is ***cytoplasm.*** It consists of clear jelly like fluid called ***cytosol* or *intracellular fluid*** in which different ***organelles* and *microfilaments*** and microtubules are found. The cytosol consists mainly of water in which various molecules are dissolved or suspended. These molecules include proteins, fats and carbohydrates as well as sodium, potassium, calcium and chloride ions. Many of the reactions that take place in the cell occur in the cytosol. There are large particles of fat, glycogen and melanin that have been produced by the cell. They are often large enough to be seen with the light microscope. For example the cells of adipose tissue (fat layer under the skin) contain fat that takes up most of the cell. The main organelles in the cell are the ***endoplasmic reticulum, mitochondrion, golgi complex, ribosomes*** **and** ***lysosomes***.

iii. Endoplasmic Reticulum (ER)

The **endoplasmic reticulum** is a network of sacs that manufactures, processes and transports chemical compounds for use inside and outside of the cell. The **endoplasmic reticulum** *(ER)* form channels throughout the cytoplasm from the nucleus to the plasma membrane. It is connected to the double layered nuclear envelope, providing a connection between nucleus and cytoplasm. Endoplasmic reticulum modifies proteins produced in the ribosomes. There are two types of ER as smooth ER and rough ER. In **smooth ER** fats are made and chemicals like alcohol, pesticides and carcinogenic molecules are inactivated. Rough ER has ribosomes attached to its surface. The function of the **rough ER** is to make proteins that are modified, stored and transported by the ER.

iv. Mitochondria

Mitochondria are found in the cytoplasm of every eukaryotic cell. In the animal cell, they are the main power generators, converting oxygen and nutrients into energy. Mitochondria produce the cell's energy and called *powerhouses* of the cell. They make energy by burning food molecules like glucose. This process is called **cellular respiration**. The reaction requires oxygen and produces carbon dioxide which is a waste product. The process is very complex and takes place in a large number of steps but the overall equation for cellular respiration is *glucose* + *oxygen* = *carbon dioxide* + *water* + *energy*. It is to note that cellular respiration is different from respiration or breathing. Breathing means the process by which air is drawn into and expelled from the lungs. Breathing is necessary to supply cells with the oxygen required by the mitochondria and to remove carbon dioxide produced as a waste product of cellular respiration. Active cells like muscle, liver, kidney and sperm cells have large numbers of mitochondria.

v. Golgi apparatus

Golgi apparatus is the central delivery system for the cell. It is group of flattened sacs arranged like a stack of bowls that modifies proteins and fats built in the endoplasmic reticulum and prepare them for export to the outside of the cell. The golgi also helps in packaging and shipping proteins to other parts of the cell or out of the cell. Golgi bodies are found near the nucleus and consist of flattened membranes stacked on top of each other like a pile of plates.

vi. Lysosomes

Lysosomes are large vesicles that contain digestive enzymes. The main function of lysosome is digestion. Lysosomes break down cellular waste products and debris from outside the cell into simple compounds, which are transferred to the cytoplasm as new cell building materials by phagocytosis or pinocytosis. They also break down harmful cell products and waste materials, cellular debris and foreign invaders such as bacteria and then force them out of the cell.

vii. Nucleus

The ***nucleus*** is the largest and highly specialized structure of cell that serves as the information and administrative center of cell. It is a spherical or oval body that contains the ***chromosomes.*** Nucleus is called brain or control center of the cell. Nucleus contains a liquid known as karyolymph, a ***nucleolus*** and chromatin. Chromatin contains deoxyribonucleic acids (*DNA*), that carriers genetic information. Two strands of DNA forming a double helix. Both the strands are twisted and folded to form *chromosomes*. It contains DNA, which makes up genes. The DNA gets *transcribed* or copied onto messenger RNA. That messenger carries a copy of the genes orders for protein synthesis. A double membrane similar in structure to the plasma membrane called *nuclear membrane or nuclear envelope* surrounds the nucleus. The *nuclear envelope* merge at the nuclear pores. Pores in this nuclear membrane allow communication between the nucleus and the cytoplasm. Within the nucleus one or more spherical bodies of darker material is seen which are called *nucleoli.* Nucleoli are made up of RNA and their role is to make new ribosomes.

viii. Ribosomes

Ribosomes are tiny spherical organelles that make proteins by joining amino acids together. Many ribosomes are found free in the cytosol, while others are attached to the rough endoplasmic reticulum.All living cells contain ribosomes which are composed of approximately 60 percent RNA and 40 percent protein. In eukaryotes, ribosomes are made of four strands of RNA. In prokaryotes, they consist of three strands of RNA. Ribosomes are the protein factories which follow instructions from messenger RNA and synthesize specific proteins.

ix. Centrioles

Centrioles are self replicating organelles made up of nine bundles of microtubules and are found only in animal cells. Centrioles are very important in cellular division.

x. Chloroplast

Chloroplasts are the structures which allow plants to trap sunlight and carry out photosynthesis.

xi. Cilia and Flagella

For single celled eukaryotes, **cilia and flagella** are essential for locomotion of individual organisms. Most eukaryotic cells lack flagella. Cilia are especially notable on the single celled protozoans, where they beat in synchrony to move the cells through water. In multicellular organisms, cilia function to move fluid or materials.

xii. Microtubules

These are straight, hollow cylinders, composed of *tubulin* protein and are found throughout the cytoplasm of all eukaryotic cells. Microtubules function as the framework along which organelles and vesicles move within a cell. They are the thickest of the cytoskeleton structures. Microtubules form *mitotic spindles* that help in the process of cell division. Microtubules and microfilaments are involved in establishing the shape or movements of the cytoskeleton the internal structure of the cell.

xiii. Microfilaments

Microfilaments are solid rods made of globular proteins called actin. These filaments are primarily structural in function and are an important component of the cytoskeleton. Microfilaments provide mechanical support to cell that determines the shape of cell. They are made of protein actin and are involved in cell motility. They are found in almost every cell, but are predominant in muscle cells.

xiv. Peroxisomes

There are several types of microbodies present in cell but peroxisomes are the most common. **Peroxisomes** are organelles in which oxygen is used to oxidize substances, breaking down lipids and detoxifying certain chemicals.

xv. Vacuoles

These are the small spaces in the cytoplasm that serve to carry materials to cell membrane to discharge outside of the cell. **Vacuoles** are formed during endocytosis when portions of the cell membrane are pinched off.

Questions

1. **What is the function of different organelles in eukaryotic cell?**
2. **What is the difference between animal cell and plant cell?**

Choose the Best Answer

1. **Basic unit of life is**

   a) Atom b) Water
   c) Cell d) Chemical level of organization

2. **Steroid hormones easliy pass through plasma membrane by simple diffusion because they are**

   a) Hydrophilic
   b) Water soluble
   c) Contain carbon and hydrogen
   d) Lipid soluble

3. **The body systems which coordinate all other body systems to maintain homoeostasis are**

   a) Cardiovascular and nervous systems
   b) Endocrine and nervous systems
   c) Digestive and cardiovascular systems
   d) Endocrine and urinary systems

4. **Glycogen is a**

   a) Carbohydrate b) Nucleic acid
   c) Lipid d) Protein

5. **An example of a secondary structure of a protein is**
   a) Globular shape
   b) Sequence of amino acids
   c) Arrangement of mulitple polypeptide chains
   d) Coil

6. **Extracellular fluid includes**
   a) Cytoplasm b) Plasma
   c) Interstitial fluid d) b and c

7. **Majority of body fluid is part of the**
   a) Intracellular fluid b) Extracellular fluid
   c) Both d) None

8. **The most common type of chemical bond in biological molecules is**
   a) Ionic b) Hydrogen
   c) Covalent d) Peptide

9. **Which is a polysaccaride**
   a) Sugar b) Glucose
   c) Lactose d) Glycogen

10. **Building blocks of lipids is**
    a) Amino acids b) Monosaccharide
    c) Fatty acid and glycerol d) Waxes

11. **Which is not related to lipid**
    a) Waxes b) Polysaccharide
    c) Steroid d) Fat

12. **Which organell has enzymes for ATP production**
    a) Golgi apparatus b) Smooth ER
    c) Mitochondrial cristae d) Cytoplasm

13. **Red blood cells appear normal in**
    a) Isotonic solution b) Hypertonic solution
    c) Hypotonic solution d) Hyperosmotic solution

14. Small lipid-soluble molecules move in and out of cells by

a) Active transport
b) Facilitated diffusion
c) Simple diffusion
d) An energy-requiring pump

15. Facilitated diffusion

a) Involves a carrier molecule
b) Requires energy expenditure
c) Moves substances against concentration gradient
d) None of above

16. Primary structure of a protein refers to its

a) Shape
b) Hydrogen bonding
c) Chemical properties
d) Amino acid sequence

17. Homeostasis means

a) Contributor and provider
b) Expand
c) Same or constant
d) Receiver

18. Normally pH of body fluid is

a) 7.15-7.25
b) 7.35-7.45
c) 7.00-7.35
d) 6.5-7.5

19. Sum of all chemical reactions in body is

a) Growth
b) Differentiation
c) Metabolism
d) All

20. Urge to breathe comes in response to

a) Time of last breath
b) Oxygen concentration surrounding
c) Buildup of nitrogen within blood
d) pH of blood

21. Homeostasis is maintained primarily by which mechanisms

a) Negative feedback
b) Malfunctioning control system
c) Positive feedback
d) Negative impact

22. Smallest structure which is capable of carrying out all life processes is

a) Muscle b) Tissue
c) Cell d) All

23. Body's thermostat is found at

a) Hypothalamus b) Skin
c) Liver d) kidney

24. Which system has little contribution to homeostasis of the organism

a) Urinary System b) Reproductive System
c) Respiratory System d) Nervous System

25. Diffusion of water across a semi permeable or selectively permeable membrane is termed as

a) Active transport b) Diffusion
c) Osmosis d) Endocytosis

26. Oxygen enters cell by

a) Diffusion b) Filtration
c) Osmosis d) Active transport

27. Term used to describe"cell eating" is

a) Exocytosis b) Phagocytosis
c) Pinocytosis d) Diffusion

28. Which of the following requires energy

a) Diffusion b) Osmosis
c) Active transport d) Facilitated diffusion

29. Protein synthesis occurs at

a) Mitochondria b) Lysosomes
c) Within the nucleus d) Ribosomes

30. Which of the following is not found in cell membrane

a) Cholesterol b) Phospholipids
c) Proteins d) Galactose

31. Cell is a

a) Largest living unit within body
b) Enzymes that eat bacteria
c) Fundamental units of all living things
d) All of the above

32. DNA is found on

a) Mitoconria b) Ribosomes
c) Chromosones d) Cytoplasm

33. Transcription occurs in

a) Cytoplasm b) Golgi apparatus
c) Mitochondria d) Nucleus

34. Start codon find at the beginning of each mRNA is

a) AGU b) GAU
c) UAG d) AUG

35. Mitosis cause each new cell which has

a) Twice as many chromosomes as its parent cell
b) Half as many chromosomes as its parent cell
c) Four times as many chromosomes as its parent cell
d) Same number of chromosomes as its parent cell

36. If a Cell is placed in an isotonic solution, it will

a) Shrink b) Swell
c) Neither swell nor shrink d) None

37. Homeostatic imbalance

a) Must be restored by negative feedback mechanisms
b) Is considered the cause of most diseases
c) Is when the internal conditions of body become more stable
d) Only occur when positive feedback mechanisms are overwhelmed

38. An organ is defined as a specific structure and is composed on two or more different types of

a) Molecules b) Cells
c) Systems d) Tissues

39. Two body systems that regulate homeostasis are

a) Nervous and endocrine systems
b) Cardiovascular and urinary systems
c) Cardiovascular and endocrine systems
d) Nervous and cardiovascular systems

40. Which one describes the endocrine system

a) It regulates homeostasis by means of nerve impulses
b) It absorbs nutrients
c) It contains hair, skin, and nails
d) It is made up of glands that secrete hormones

41. Body system that distributes oxygen and nutrients to cells and carries carbon dioxide and wastes away from cells is

a) Respiratory system b) Cardiovascular system
c) Endocrine system d) Urinary system

42. The body system that regulate volume and chemical composition of blood and regulate fluid and electrolyte balance is

a) Respiratory system b) Cardiovascular system
c) Endocrine system d) Urinary system

43. Which of the following are considered part as of the integumentary system?

a) Liver, stomach, and intestines
b) Brain and spinal cord
c) Hormonesecreting glands
d) Hair, skin, and nails

44. Tissue is defined as

a) Basic structural and functional unit of an organism
b) Molecules that form the body's structure
c) Group of cells and the surrounding materials that work together to perform a particular function
d) Group of related organs with a common function

45. Body systems that provides protection against disease and returns proteins and plasma to the cardiovascular system is

a) Respiratory
b) Urinary
c) Endocrine
d) Lymphatic

46. Skeletal system

a) Provides support and protection.
b) Stores minerals.
c) Assists in body movements.
d) All of the above are true.

47. Homeostasis is the condition in which body maintains

a) Lowest possible energy usage
b) Relatively stable internal environment, within limits
c) A static state with no deviation from preset points
d) A changing state, within an unlimited range

48. Anabolism is

a) Breakdown of matter
b) Expulsion of matter
c) Synthesis of matter
d) All of the above

49. Homeostasis refers to

a) Unwavering control of a physiological setpoint
b) Maintaining a stable internal environment
c) Maintaining a stable external environment
d) a and b

Answers

1. c	2. d	3. b	4. a	5. d	6. d	7. a	8. c	9. d	10. c
11. b	12. c	13. a	14. c	15. a	16. d	17. c	18. b	19. c	20. d
21. a	22. c	23. a	24. b	25. c	26. a	27. b	28. c	29. d	30.d
31. c	32. c	33. d	34. d	35. d	36. c	37. b	38. d	39. a	40.d
41. b	42. d	43. d	44. c	45. d	46. d	47. b	48. c	49. b	

□□□

CHAPTER-2

Blood and Cardiovascular System

Blood is the **connective tissue fluid** of body and considered as fluid of life because it carries oxygen from lungs to all parts of the body and CO_2 from all parts of the body to lungs. There are three classes of blood cells (corpuscles) as **erythrocytes** (red blood cells), **leucocytes** (white blood cells), **thrombocytes** (platelets). The red colour of blood is due to the hemoglobin present in the erythrocytes. All these cells are suspended in the fluid called **plasma**. Plasma is yellow to colourless depending on the quantity, species of the animal and animal's diet. The colour of plasma is mainly due to pigment called **bilirubin** although carotene and other pigments are contributing factors. Blood consists of 50 -60% of liquid (plasma) and 40-50% of solid part. When blood is centrifuged, in between plasma and RBC there is WBC. **Erythrocyte** is red blood cells (RBCs) which transport hemoglobin that inturn carry oxygen from lungs to tissue. Erythrocytes in mammals are non nucleated and non motile cells. They usually appear biconcave, circular disc with a central pale spot. The biconcavity increases surface area and decreases diffusion distance thus facilitating the exchange of oxygen and carbon dioxide carried by RBCs. Erythrocytes vary in diameter and thickness according to species and nutritional status of the animal and they are also capable of changing shape while passing through capillary. Though erythrocyte is biconcave but this concavity also varies as per species. Goat has the largest number of red blood cells per unit volume and smallest cell in diameter. **Erythropoiesis** is the process by which RBC is originated, developed and matured. In simple way it can be expressed as formation of RBCs. **Hemopoiesis** is origin, development and maturation of all blood cells. Erythropoiesis is a continuous process. Many nutrients are essential for this process. Because of continuous need to replenish RBCs, new RBCs has to form continuously. Blood cells begin their lives in the bone marrow from a single type of cell called **pluripotential hematopoietic stem cell**, from which all the cells of circulating blood are derived. The number of RBCs varies greatly among species and also within individuals of same species. Several factors affect not also erythrocytic count but also hemoglobin concentration and other blood constituents. These factors are age, sex, exercise, nutritional status, lactation, pregnancy, egg production, excitement, blood volume, stage of estrus cycle, breed, environmental temperature, altitude and other clinical factors. The percentage of blood cells are called **hematocrit** percentage. It consists of erythrocyte mass (PCV) and leucocytes. The rate at which the cells settle down is called **erythrocyte sedimentation rate (ESR).** ESR is a test of blood to determine the health status of an animal. ESR is determined by Westergren's method or Wintrobe's tube method. Normally ESR is 3-7mm/hr in male and 5-9mm/hr in female.

Hemoglobin is the pigment of erythrocytes. Synthesis of hemoglobin begins in the proerythroblast and continues in the subsequent stage of cell development. This stage of development of hemoglobin continues even into the reticulocyte stage of RBCs. The affinity of oxygen with hemoglobin in fetal blood is higher than that of adult/maternal blood. Ruminants have structurally distinct fetal hemoglobin which have higher oxygen affinity than adult hemoglobin, thereby permitting oxygen-hemoglobin affinity is higher than those of mother. Dog, horse and pig don't have structurally different hemoglobin but in these species the fetal RBCs have much lower 2,3 biphosphoglycerate (BPG) than adult RBCs, thereby creating higher oxygen affinity in fetal RBCs. Excitement may increase the hemoglobin concentration because of increased PCV and erythrocyte number per unit of volume. Hemoglobin readily combines with gas or other substances to form some products which are called derivatives of hemoglobin. These derivatives are **oxyhemoglobin, myoglobin, carbhemoglobin, carboxyhemoglobin, methemoglobin etc**. In human spleen is the important place of RBC destruction. In rabbit and gunea pig spleen is of less importance. In bird liver is the main place of RBC destruction. After hemolysis of RBC iron and globin are separated from heme. Globin is degraded into amino acids and iron is stored in macrophages in the form of ***ferritin*** and ***hemosiderin*** and then transport to plasma where it combines with plasma protein, ***apotransferrin*** to become ***transferrin.*** Transferrin is circulated to bone marrow where the iron is used for synthesis of new hemoglobin. **Anemia** means deficiency of hemoglobin in blood which can be caused by either reduction in red blood cells count and packed cell volume. Anemia can be classified by two methods as morphological classification and etiological classification. On the basis of size and hemoglobin content of RBCs the anemia is classified in to four types as **normocytic normochromic anemia, macrocytic normochromic anemia, macrocytic hypochromic anemia and microcytic hypochromic anemia.** On the basis of cause, anemia is of four types as **hemorrhagic anemia, hemolytic anemia, nutritional deficiency anemia and aplastic anemia**.

White blood cell (WBC) or leucocyte is the colourless and nucleated elements of blood. WBCs are the mobile unit of body's protective or defense system. They are formed partially in bone marrow and partially in lymph in lymph tissue. Most of the WBCs are transported to the areas of infection and inflammation. Depending on presence and absence of granules in cytoplasm the leucocytes are classified in to two types as i) **Granulocytes** (with granules) which include neutrophils, eosinophils and basophils and ii) **Agranulocytes** (without granules) which include lymphocytes and monocytes. The life span of leucocyte is not so easily measured as that of erythrocytes. The circulating blood transport the leucocytes to the site of action. The mean life span of granulocytes including the time of development in bone marrow is approximately 9 days. When granulocytes enter blood stream they are about 6 days old. **Neutrophil** plays an important role in defense of the body. **Eosinophils** normally constitute about 2-5% of blood leucocytes and plays important role in defense of body. Major function of these leucocytes are detoxification, disintegration and removal of foreign proteins. **Basophils** in blood are similar to the tissue mast cells located immediately outside many of the capillaries in body. Both basophils and mast cells secrete heparin that prevent blood coagulation. **Monocytes** plays important role in defense of body. Along with neutrophills, monocyte constitute the first line of defense. Like neutrophills, monocytes are motile and phagocytic. **Lymphocytes** plays important role in immunity. Functionally lymphocytes are classified into two types as T-lymphocytes and B-lymphocytes. T-lymphocytes are responsible for cellular immunity B-lymphocytes are responsible for humeral immunity. **Platelets or thrombocytes** are small, colourless, round or rod shaped bodies in blood of mammals. Platelets are responsible or having role in **blood clotting, hemostasis**

(blood loss), repairing of ruptured blood vessels and helps in **defense mechanism** by encircling the foreign body and kill them by the process of phagocytosis.

Hemostasis means prevention of blood loss or stoppage of bleeding. When a blood vessel is ruptured or injured the injury initiates a series of reactions or mechanisms that results hemostasis. These mechanisms are i) vasoconstriction ii) formation of platelet plug iii) coagulation of blood iv) growth of fibrous tissue into blood clot to close the hole in vessel permanently. Coagulation of blood occurs through series of reactions due to activation of group of substances called **clotting factors**. These series of reactions involves three essential steps as i) formation of prothrombin activator ii) conversion of prothrombin to thrombin catalyzed by prothrombin activator and iii) conversion of fibrinogen to fibrin catalyzed by thrombin. Prothrombin activator are generally formed in two ways as extrinsic pathway and intrinsic pathway. Extrinsic pathway begins with trauma to vascular wall and surrounding tissue where as intrinsic pathway begins in the blood itself. In both this pathways different plasma proteins i.e clotting factors plays important role. Most of these factors are in inactive form of proteolytic enzymes but when they are converted to active form their enzymatic actions cause the successive cascading reactions of clotting process. There are thirteen clotting factors are identified which plays their role in clot formation.

Cardio vascular system comprises of heart and blood vessels. Heart is the central pump and blood vessels are the series of distributing and collecting tubes. Mainly blood vessels are categorized into 3 groups as i) **arteries:** These are the conducting systems that distribute blood from heart to organs and tissue, ii) **arterioles and capillaries:** These include micro circulation and concerned with blood distribution and diffusion within organ and tissues and iii) **Veins:** These are the conducting system that collects blood from the organs and tissues to heart. **Heart** is two chambers pump composed of an atrium and ventricle. Atria acts as a primer pump. Blood normally flow continually from the great veins into atria. About 75% of the blood flows directly through the atria into the ventricles even before atria contract. Ventricle supplies blood either through the pulmonary circulation by right ventricle or through peripheral circulation by left ventricle. Ventricle makes up most of the heart weight. The two atria of heart are separated from each other by fibrous septum called **inter atrial septum**. Two ventricles are separated from each other by muscular septum called **inter ventricular septum.** There are four valves in mammalian heart. Out of these four valves two are in between atria and ventricle called **atrio-ventricular valve** (AV valves). The other two valves are **semilunar valves** at the opening of blood vessels arises from ventricles. These semilunar valves are **aortic** and **pulmonary** semilunar valve. The left AV valve is otherwise called as **mitral valve or bicuspid valve.** It is formed by two valvular cusps or flaps. Right AV valve is called as **tricuspid valve** and it is formed by three cusps. The aortic and pulmonary semilunar valve function quite differently from AV valve. The semilunar valves are present at the opening of the aorta and pulmonary artery and are known as **aortic valve** and **pulmonary valve** respectively. Both the semilunar valves are similar in structure and each has three flaps. These valves open towards aorta and pulmonary artery and prevent back flow of blood into ventricle. These semilunar valves prevent back flow of blood from aorta and pulmonary artery into ventricle during diastole. Heart is made up of three layers of tissues as **pericardium** the outer layer, **myocardium** the middle layer and **endocardium** the inner layer. Heart is consisting of special system that generates rhythmical electrical impulses to cause rhythmical contraction of heart muscle and conducting these impulses rapidly through the heart. Specialized excitatory and conducting system of heart that control cardiac contractions are sinoatrial node (SA) node, intermodal fibers, atrio ventricular node, atrio ventricular (AV) bundle, purkinje fibers. Cardiac muscle is striated in the same way as skeletal muscle. Cardiac muscle has myofibrils that contain myocin and actin filaments those are identical to skeletal muscle fibers. These filaments lie side by side and slide along one another during contraction in the same manner as occurs in skeletal muscle. The cell membrane that separate individual cardiac muscle cell from one another is called **intercalated disc**. Cardiac muscle fiber are made up of many individual cells connected in series with one another. Heart is consisting of two syncytium as **atrial syncytium** and **ventricular syncytium.** The action potential of skeletal muscle is caused entirely by sudden opening of large number of fast sodium channels. These channels are called fast as it remains open for 10,000th of a second and then suddenly close but in cardiac muscle the action potential is caused by the opening of two types of channels. They are i) Fast sodium channel like in skeletal muscle ii) By slow calcium channels called Calcium-Sodium channels. Each heart beat consists of two major period called systole and diastole. During systole there is contraction of cardiac muscle and pumping of blood from heart.

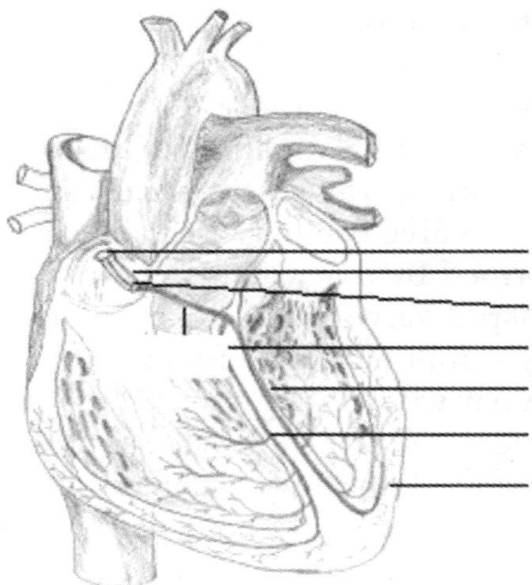

Heart

During diastole there is relaxation of cardiac muscle and filling of blood. Various changes or events occurs in different chambers of heart during each heart beat. These changes are repeated during each heart beat in a cyclic manner. So the changes or events that occur from beginning of one heart beat to beginning of next is called **cardiac cycle**. The mechanical activities of heart during each cardiac cycle produces sounds called **heart sound**. Normally the heart sounds are produced due to movement of cardiac muscle, valves of the heart and by passing of blood through chamber of heart. These sounds can be heard by stethoscope and recorded graphically. There are **four heart sounds** produces during each cardiac cycle. The **first and second heart sounds** are prominent and sounds as 'lub' and 'dub'. The 'lub' sound is produced due to closure of AV valve at the beginning of systole and the sound 'dub' is associated with the closure of semilunar valve at the end of systole and onset of diastole. The **third heart sound** is a weak, rumbling sound heard occasionally at the beginning of middle third of diastole during rapid filling period of cardiac cycle. Normally this third heart sound is not audible by stethoscope. It can be heard by microphone. **Fourth heart sound** is produced during atrial systole in some cases and can be recorded graphically by phonocardiogram. When cardiac impulse passes through heart there is passes of electrical currents from heart to surrounding tissues. These small currents produced can be recorded by using suitable electrodes by placing them on body on opposite site of heart. Recording of these currents is called

electrocardiogram *or ECG.* The normal electrocardiogram is composed of P wave, QRS complex and T wave. QRS complex is often composed of three separate waves as 'Q' wave, 'R' wave and 'S' wave but not always. **P wave** is caused by electrical potential generated when the atria depolarize at the beginning of the atrial contraction. *QRS wave* is generated when the ventricle depolarize at the beginning of the ventricular contraction. **T wave** is the potential generated due to repolarization of ventricle. The means by which blood is pumped by the heart is regulated are i) **intrinsic cardiac regulation of pumping** in response to changes in volume of blood flowing in to heart and ii) control of heart rate and strength of heart pumping by autonomic nervous system called **extrinsic regulation of pumping**. The intrinsic ability of heart to adapt to increasing volumes of inflowing blood is called **Frank starling mechanism** of the heart. **Extrinsic regulation of heart pumping** is controlled by autonomic nervous system through sympathetic and parasympathetic nerves.

Short Questions and Answers

Blood

1. What is Composition and function of blood?

Ans. Blood is the *connective tissue fluid* of body and considered as fluid of life because it carries oxygen from lungs to all parts of the body and CO_2 from all parts of the body to lungs. There are three classes of blood cells (corpuscles) as **erythrocytes** (red blood cells), **leucocytes** (white blood cells), **thrombocytes** (platelets).The red colour of blood is due to the hemoglobin present in the erythrocytes. All these cells are suspended in the fluid called **plasma**. Plasma is yellow to colourless depending on the quantity, species of the animal and animal's diet. Blood consists of 50 -60% of liquid (plasma) and 40-50% of solid part. When blood is centrifuged in between plasma and RBC there is WBC.

2. What is difference between serum and plasma?

Ans. After coagulation the blood clot retracts from a clear watery fluid called **serum**. Serum is similar to plasma except the **fibrinogen** and other clotting factors. In adult animal plasma is 91-92% water and 8-9% solid.

3. What is Anticoagulants? Name some anticoagulants.

Ans. Anticoagulants are substances that interfere with the clotting process. **Heparin** a conjugated polysaccharide is the **natural anticoagulant** produced by the basophills in the blood and mast cell throughout the body. From mast cells of connective tissue heparin is also released. Concentration of 0.2 mg (20 units) of heparin per ml of blood is used as anticoagulant. One unit of heparin is approximately 0.01mg of heparin sodium. Other anticoagulants used are sodium, potassium and ammonium salt of oxalate and fluride. Chelating agents like ethylene diamine tetra acetic acid (EDTA) are also used for hematological studies. Heparin and EDTA are two anticoagulants which keeps the size of erythrocytes constant when recommended concentration are used in hematological procedure. Out of this two EDTA is the preferred anticoagulant for blood morphological studies.

4. What is erythropoiesis?

Ans. It is the process by which RBC is originated, developed and matured. In simple way it can be expressed as formation of RBCs. **Hemopoiesis** is origin, development and maturation of all blood cells. Erythropoiesis is a continuous process. Many nutrients are essential for this process. Erythropoietic cells are the most rapidly growing and reproducing cells in the entire body. Blood cells begin their lives in the bone marrow from a single type of cell called **pluripotential hematopoietic stem cell**. These stem cells goes for successive divisions like **intermediate stage cells** and **committed stem cells** stage to form different circulating blood cells.

5. What is Composition of erythrocyte?

Ans. Erythrocyte in adult animal contain 62-72% of water and 35% of solids. **Hemoglobin** constitute about 95% of the solids. The remaining solids are proteins in stroma and cell membrane, lipids such as phospholipids (lecithin, cephalin, sphingomyelin), cholesterol, natural fat, vitamins, carbohydrates (glucose) for energy, enzymes like choline esterase, phosphatase, carbonic anhydrase, peptides and those concern with glycolysis and minerals like phosphorous, sulpher, chlorine, magnesium, potassium and sodium.

Potassium is the principal cation of erythrocyte in some species, like pig, chicken and some breeds of sheep where as in other animals like cat, dog, cow, goat and sheep the principal cation is sodium. Chlorine is the principal anion in all species. It is well documented that domestic animals exhibit genetic differences in the potassium content of erythrocyte.

6. What is packed cell volume (PCV)?

Ans. The components of blood are separated according to specific gravity by centrifugation. PCV is expressed as percentage in volume of packed cells in whole blood after centrifugation. The percentage of blood cells are called **hematocrit** percentage. It consists of erythrocyte mass (PCV) and leucocytes. The PCV occupied lowest part of the hematocrit, leucocyte become a narrow band after centrifugation and placed above PCV and referred as **buffy coat**. PCV is often referred as hematocrit but more correctly it is component of hematocrit. PCV is approximately three times more than hemoglobin concentration. In animal PCV ranges from 25-45%.

7. What is erythrocyte sedimentation rate (ESR)?

Ans. It is the speed at which erythrocyte is settle down and this value is expressed in mm/hr. The rate at which the cells settle down is called **erythrocyte sedimentation rate (ESR).** ESR is a test of blood to determine the health status of an animal. ESR is determined by Westergren's method or Wintrobe's tube method. Normally ESR is 3-7mm/hr in male and 5-9mm/hr in female. ESR is affected by age, sex, pregnancy etc. ESR is less in children and infants. Females have more ESR than male. ESR is increased upto 35mm/hr during pregnancy. ESR is increased in disease like tuberculosis, anemia (except sickle cell anemia), malignant tumor, rheumatoid arthritis and liver diseases where as ESR is decreased in allergic condition, sickle cell anemia, shock, polycythemia etc.

8. How hemoglobin is synthesized?

Ans. Synthesis of hemoglobin begins in the proerythroblast and continues in the subsequent stage of cell development. Basic chemical steps for the formation of hemoglobin are

i) Succinyl CoA forms in the kreb's cycle binds to glycine to form Pyrrole molecule.

ii) Four pyrrole molecules combines to form protoporphyrin IX which combines with iron to form hemoglobin

iii) Finally each heme molecules combine with a long polypeptide chain a globin synthesized by ribosomes and forming a subunit of hemoglobin called a hemoglobin chain. Each chain has a molecular weight of 16,000. Four of these chains in turn binds together loosely to form whole hemoglobin molecule.

9. What are the derivatives of hemoglobin?

Ans. Hemoglobin readily combines with gas or other substances to form some products which are called derivatives of hemoglobin. The derivatives are

i) Oxyhemoglobin

Hemoglobin has physiological relationship with oxygen when hemoglobin combines with oxygen. Oxyhemoglobin is an unstable compound and this combination is irreversible. When saturated with oxygen, 1 gram hemoglobin carries about 1.34 ml of oxygen so as a result 15gm of hemoglobin in 100ml of blood may carry approximately 20 ml of oxygen.

ii) Myoglobin

It is also called as **muscle hemoglobin**. It is true hemoglobin which is composed of heme an only one peptide chain. The heme is identical to that of blood hemoglobin but globin of blood hemoglobin differs globin muscle hemoglobin by amino acid contents. Myoglobin has greater affinity for oxygen than blood hemoglobin.

iii) Carbhemoglobin

It is the hemoglobin in combination with carbon dioxide. The affinity of hemoglobin for CO_2 is 20 times more than oxygen. Carbon monoxide prevents hemoglobin from being a carrier of oxygen, thus it interferes with hemoglobin supplying oxygen to tissue.

iv) **Carboxyhemoglobin**

The combination of hemoglobin with carbon monoxide produces carboxyhemoglobin. Affinity of hemoglobin for carbon monoxide is more than 200 times greater than for oxygen thus interferes with hemoglobin supplying oxygen to the tissue. Carboxyhemoglobin is bright cherry red in colour.

v) **Methemoglobin**

It is the derivative of hemoglobin that is formed by the oxidation of ferrous iron of hemoglobin to the ferric state. Methemoglobin is the true oxide of hemoglobin but oxyhemoglobin is an oxygenated derivative. Methemoglobin is otherwise called as **ferrihemoglobin.** Many chemical substances like nitrites, aminophenols, sulphonamides etc and certain oxidizing agents promotes the conversion of hemoglobin to methemoglobin.

vi) **Sulphe hemoglobin and nitrous oxide hemoglobin**

Sulphe hemoglobin is formed by combination of hemoglobin with hydrogen sulphide where as nitrous oxide hemoglobin is formed when hemoglobin is combines with nitrous oxide.

10. What is mean corpuscular volume (MCV)?

Ans. It is average volume of a single RBC and it is expressed in cubic micron (cuμ). The normal MCV is 90 cuμ. When MCV is increased the cell is called **macrocytic** but when it is decreased it is called **microcytic** and when MCV is normal it called **normocytic**. MCV can be calculated by mathematical formula as **MCV = PCV(%) x 10 / TEC (10^6/μl).**

11. What is mean corpuscular hemoglobin (MCH)?

Ans. This is defined as the amount of hemoglobin present in one RBC. It is expressed micro micro gram or pico gram. The normal MCH in haman is 30 pico gram. When MCH is normal it is called as **normochromic**. MCH can be calculated by mathematical formula as **MCH = Hb Conc. (g/dl) x 10 / TEC (10^6/μl).**

12. What is mean corpuscular hemoglobin concentration (MCHC)?

Ans. This is the concentration of hemoglobin in one RBC. It is the amount of hemoglobin expressed in relation to the volume of one RBC. So here the unit of expression is percentage. Normal value of MCHC is 30%. This MCHC value is important to diagnose anemia. **MCHC** represents indirectly the colour index of erythrocytes. When MCHC is normal it means **normochromic** cells where as lesser MCHC means **hypochromic** cells and higher MCHC means **hyperchromic** cells. MCHC can be calculated by mathematical formula as **MCHC = Hb Conc. (g/dl) x 100 / PCV(%).**

13. What is polycythemia?

Ans. When tissue becomes hypoxic due to less oxygen in breathed air because of high altitudes or due to failure of oxygen delivery to tissue such as cardiac failure then the blood forming organs automatically produce **large quantities of extra red blood cells**. This condition is called **polycythemia**. Polycythemia is of two types as i) Primary polycythemia and ii) Secondary polycythemia

i) Primary polycythemia

This condition is otherwise called as **polycythemia vera**. It is a disease in which there is persistent increase in RBC count. In this condition PCV (hematocrit) becomes 60-70% instead 40-45% in normal. There is increase in blood volume as of which the entire vascular system becomes intensively engorged.

ii) Secondary polycythemia

When the tissue becomes hypoxic because of too little oxygen in breathed air due to high altitudes or because of failure of oxygen delivery to tissue such as cardiac failure, the blood forming organs automatically produce large quantities of extra RBCs. This condition is called **secondary polycythemia**. In this condition RBCs count increases 30% above normal. Common type of secondary polycythemia is called **physiological polycythemia** that occurs when one live at high altitude of 14,000-17,000 feet where the atmospheric oxygen is low.

14. What is anemia?

Ans. **Anemia** means deficiency of hemoglobin in blood which can be caused by either reduction in red blood cells count and packed cell volume. Anemia can be classified by two methods as morphological classification and etiological classification. **Morphological classification** is on the basis of size and hemoglobin content of RBCs and include normocytic normochromic anemia, macrocytic normochromic anemia, macrocytic hypochromic anemia and microcytic hypochromic anemia where as **etiological classification** is on the basis of cause and include hemorrhagic anemia, hemolytic anemia, nutritional deficiency anemia and aplastic anemia.

15. What is white blood cell?

Ans. **White blood cell (WBC)** or **leucocyte** is the colourless and nucleated elements of blood. WBCs are the mobile unit of body's protective or defense system. They are formed partially in bone marrow and partially in lymph in lymph tissue. Most of the WBCs are transported to the areas of infection and inflammation. Depending on presence and absence of granules in cytoplasm the leucocytes are classified in to two types as i) **Granulocytes** (with granules) which include neutrophils, eosinophils and basophils and ii) **Agranulocytes** (without granules) which include lymphocytes and monocytes. Leucocytes are much less numerous than erythrocytes in circulating blood. Erythrocyte function in blood stream while leucocyte carry their function predominantly in tissue.

16. What are the functions of white blood cells?

Ans. **Neutrophil** plays an important role in defense of the body. Neutrophils and monocytes provide the first line of defense against the invading microorganism. Neutrophils contain enzymes like protease, myeloperoxidase, elastage and metallo proteins. **Eosinophils** helps in detoxification, disintegration and removal of foreign proteins. **Basophils** play important role in healing process after inflammation and allergic reaction. **Monocytes** plays important role in defense of body. Along with neutrophills, monocyte constitute the first line of defense. Like neutrophills, monocytes are motile and phagocytic. **Lymphocytes** plays important role in immunity. Functionally lymphocytes are classified into two types as T-lymphocytes and B-lymphocytes. T-lymphocytes are responsible for cellular immunity B-lymphocytes are responsible for humeral immunity.

17. What are platelets and its function?

Ans. **Platelets** or **thrombocytes** are small, colourless, round or rod shaped bodies in blood of mammals. Normally platelets are spherical or rod shaped and become oval or disc shaped when inactivated. Platelets are formed in fetal liver, spleen and bone marrow. In adult principal site for platelet formation is bone marrow. Lungs are also source of platelets. Platelets are responsible or having role in b**lood clotting, hemostasis (blood loss), repairing of ruptured blood vessels** and **defense mechanism by** encircling the foreign body and kill them by the process of phagocytosis.

18. What is erythroblastosis fetalis ?

Ans. When a Rh - mother carries a Rh + fetus, then the first child escapes the complication of Rh incompatibility. This is because Rh antigen can not pass from fetal blood into mother's blood through placental barrier or it may also be explained that even if Rh antigen goes to mother's blood it does not develop sufficient anti-Rh agglutinins to cause any harm. But for subsequent pregnancy cause sufficient anti-Rh agglutinins to cause agglutination of fetal blood and hemolysis that leads to death of fetus called **erythroblastosis fetalis**. However about 3% of second Rh+ babies exhibit sign of erythroblastosis fetalis and about 10% of third baby exhibit the disease and these incidence rises progressively with subsequent pregnancies.

19. What is hemostasis?

Ans. **Hemostasis** means prevention of blood loss or stoppage of bleeding. When a blood vessel is ruptured or injured the injury initiates a series of reactions or mechanisms that results hemostasis. These mechanisms are i) vasoconstriction ii) formation of platelet plug iii) coagulation of blood iv) growth of fibrous tissue into blood clot to close the hole in vessel permanently.

20. What is general mechanism of blood coagulation?

Ans. Coagulation of blood occurs through series of reactions due to activation of group of substances called **clotting factors**. These series of reactions involves three essential steps as i) Formation of prothrombin activator ii) conversion of prothrombin to thrombin catalyzed by prothrombin activator and iii) conversion of fibrinogen to fibrin catalyzed by thrombin.

21. What are clotting factors?

Ans. Coagulation of blood occurs through series of reactions due to activation of group of substances called **clotting factors**. There are thirteen clotting factors are identified which plays their role in clot formation. These clotting factors are :

Clotting factors	**Name**
Factor I	Fibrinogen
Factor II	Prothrombin
Factor III	Thromboplastin
Factor IV	Calcium
Factor V	Proacclerin, Labile factor
Factor VI	– – – – –
Factor VII	Proconvertin, serum prothrombin conversion accelerator (SPCA), stable factor
Factor VIII	Anti hemophilic factor (AHF), Anti hemophilic globulin (AHG), Anti hemophilic factor A
Factor IX	Christmas factor, Plasma thromboplastin component (PTC), Anti hemophilic factor B
Factor X	Stuart factor

Factor XI	Plasma thrombo plastin antecedent (PTA), Anti hemophilic factor C
Factor XII	Hageman factor
Factor XIII	Fibrin stabilizing factor

22. What is extrinsic pathway of prothrombin activator formation?

Ans. The extrinsic pathway to initiate the formation of prothrombin activator begins with a traumatized vascular wall or traumatized extravascular tissue that comes in contact with blood. The steps include are

i) Release of tissue thromboplastin (Factor III)

Traumatized tissue release a complex of several factor called tissue thromboplastin (Factor III) or tissue factor. This factor consists of proteins, phospholipids and lipoproteins which acts as proteolytic enzymes.

ii) Activation of factor X

Tissue thromboplastin in combination with Factor VII and calcium ion act enzymatically and activate factor X.

iii) Formation of prothrombin activator

Activated factor X (Xa) combine immediately with tissue phospholipid which are part of tissue factor and also with additional phospholipid released from platelet as well as with factor V form a complex called prothrombin activator. Factor V is activated by thrombin which is formed from prothrombin. This factor V accelerates the formation of prothrombin activator and other process of blood clot. This effect of thrombin is called positive feed back effect.

23. What is intrinsic pathway for formation of prothrombin activator?

Ans. Intrinsic mechanism to initiate the formation of prothrombin activator begins with trauma to blood itself or exposure of blood to collagen from traumatized blood vessel wall. The steps are :

i) Activation of factor XII

Trauma to blood or exposure of blood to vascular wall collagen alter clotting factor XII. When factor XII comes in contact with collagen it becomes activated called activated factor XII (XIIa) which is a proteolytic enzyme.

ii) Activation of factor XI

Activated factor XII acts enzymatically on factor XI and activate this factor in presence of high molecular weight kinogen and prekallikrein

iii) Activation of factor IX

Activated factor XI (XIa) acts enzymatically on factor IX to activate this.

iv) Activation of factor X

Activated factor IX (IXa) in presence of factor VIII, calcium and thromboplastin activate factor X.

v) Formation of prothrombin activator

Activated factor X (Xa) combines with factor V, platelets and tissue phospholipids form a complex called prothrombin activator. This steps in intrinsic pathway is similar to that of extrinsic pathway.

24. Why blood don't clot inside blood vessel?

Ans. The most important factor to prevent clotting in the normal vascular system are :

i) Smoothness of endothelial surface that prevents contact activation of intrinsic clotting mechanism.

ii) There is presence of layer of mucopolysaccharide called **glycocalyx** on the endothelium which repeals clotting factors and platelets that prevents clotting.

iii) **Thrombomodulin** an endothelial bound protein binds with thrombin that slow down the clotting process. Thrombomodulin -thrombin complex also activates a plasma protein, protein C that acts as an anticoagulant by inactivating activated factor V and factor VIII.

iv) Presence of a natural anticoagulant known as **heparin** in blood which is a highly negative charged conjugated polysaccharide which when combines with antithrombin III then effectiveness of antithrombin III in removing thrombin increases. The complex of heparin and antithrombin III removes several other activated coagulation factor in addition to thrombin that enhance the effectiveness of anticoagulation.

v) While clot forming goes on, about 80-90% of thrombin is formed from prothrombin that get adsorbed to the fibrin fiber. This helps preventing the spread of thrombin, **therefore prevents the spread of clot**. The thrombin that does not adsorb to fibrin fiber combines with antithrombin III that blocks the effect of thrombin on fibrinogen and prevent clot.

25. What is bleeding time?

Ans. It is the time in minute require for bleeding to stops. Bleeding time is measure of platelet function. Bleeding time normally lasts for 1-6 minute. This time depends on the depth of wound. Lack of any one of the clotting factor can prolong the bleeding time but bleeding time specially prolonged by lack of platelets.

26. What is clotting time?

Ans. It is the time in minute required for the formation of fibrin strands. Clotting time reflects the activity of various coagulation factors.

27. What is prothrombin time?

Ans. It is the time required for coagulation to takes place. Prothrombin time gives indication of the quantity of prothrombin in blood.

28. What is Immunity?

Ans. Ability of body against the pathogenic agents like bacteria, virus, toxic substances etc is called as **immunity.** Immunity is of two types as **innate immunity** and **acquired immunity. Innate immunity** is other wise called as **natural immunity**.

It is present from birth which resist the entry of microorganism in to the body. **Acquired immunity** is the resistance developed in the body against any specific foreign body like bacteria, virus, toxic substances etc. When body get exposed to this factor. Lymphocytes are responsible for this type of immunity. Acquired immunity is other wise called as **adaptive immunity.**

Cardiovascular System

1. What is function of arteries?

Ans. Arteries are the conducting systems that distribute blood from heart to organs and tissue.

2. What is function of veins?

Ans. These are the conducting system that collects blood from the organs and tissues to heart.

3. What is function of arterioles and capillaries?

Ans. These include micro circulation and concerned with blood distribution and diffusion within organ and tissues.

4. What are the major divisions of cardio vascular system?

Ans. Major divisions of cardio vascular system are

i) **Distribution system** that include heart, arteries and arterioles

ii) **Distribution and perfusion system** that include arteries, arterioles and capillaries

iii) **Collecting system** that include venules, veins and heart

5. What is function of atria?

Ans. Atria is principally function as a weak primer pump for the ventricle helping to move the blood into the ventricle. Blood normally flow continually from the great veins into atria. About 75% of the blood flows directly through the atria into the ventricles even before atria contract. Then atrial contraction causes an additional 25% filling the ventricle.

6. What is function of ventricle?

Ans. Ventricle supplies blood either through the pulmonary circulation by right ventricle or through peripheral circulation by left ventricle. Ventricle makes up most of the heart weight.

7. What are the valves present in heart?

Ans. Valves of heart are made in such a way that it permits the flow of blood to heart in one direction only. There are four valves in mammalian heart. Out of these four valves two are in between atria and ventricle called **atrio-ventricular valve** (AV valves). The other two valves are **semilunar valves** at the opening of blood vessels arise from ventricles. These semilunar valves are **aortic** and **pulmonary** semilunar valve.

8. What are bicuspid and tricuspid valve?

Ans. The left **Atrio-ventricular valve** is otherwise called as **mitral valve or bicuspid valve**. It is formed by two valvular cusps or flaps. Right AV valve is called as **tricuspid valve** and it is formed by three cusps. The cusp of the valve are attached to the papillary muscles by means of **chordate tendinae**. Papillary muscles arises from inner surface of ventricles. The papillary muscles play an important role in closure of cusps and also prevent back flow of blood from ventricle to atria during ventricular contraction.

9. What are semilunar valves?

Ans. There are two semilunar valves in heart. The semilunar valves are present at the opening of the aorta and pulmonary artery and are known as **aortic valve** and **pulmonary valve** respectively. Both the semilunar valves are similar in structure and each has three flaps. These valves open towards aorta and pulmonary artery and prevent back flow of blood into ventricle. These semilunar valves prevent back flow of blood from aorta and pulmonary artery into ventricle during diastole.

10. What are Cardiac layers?

Ans. Heart is made up of three layers of tissues as **pericardium** the outer layer, **myocardium** the middle layer and **endocardium** the inner layer.

11. What are the muscle fibers forming contractile unit of heart?

Ans. Cardiac muscle fiber is involuntary where as skeletal muscle fiber is voluntary. Contractile unit of cardiac muscle fiber contain **actin, myosin, troponin** and **tropomyosin** just like skeletal muscle fiber. A special membrane junction that connects the two adjacent cells in cardiac muscle fiber is **intercalated disc.** This disc play important role during contraction of muscle by pulling muscle fibers with one another.

12. What are the functional specializations of intercalated disc?

Ans. Intercalated disc have three types of functional specialization as

i) **Macula adherens or desmosomes:** These electron dense round bodies appear to weld the sarcolemma of adjacent fibers together.

ii) **Fascia adherens or intermediate junction:** This structure is generally larger than macula adherens and occupies the major part of the transverse segments of the intercalated disc. Fascia adherens provides adhesion between adjacent cells thus allows the transmission of contractile force from cell to cell.

iii) **Nexus:** Nexus is the tight or gap junction found on the lateral portion of the disc. The plasma membrane of one cell comes in contact with that of an adjoining cell at the nexus. Nexus serve as the low resistance pathway for electrical conduction between the cells. Because of the gap junction all the cardiac muscle fibers acts like a **syncytium**. Heart is consisting of two syncytium as **atrial syncytium** and **ventricular syncytium**. These two are connected by a thick non conducting fibrous ring called **atrio-ventricular ring**.

13. What are the muscle fiber forming pace maker of heart?

Ans. Some of the muscle fiber of heart are modified into a specialized structure called **pacemaker**. Pacemaker generate the impulses for heart beat normally. Sinoatrial node (SA node) is the pacemaker in animal heart. SA node is present in right atrium just below the opening of the superior venacava. **Lewis Thomas** in 1918 named SA node as pace maker. Even though parts of heart like AV node, atria and ventricle produce impulses but SA node is called pace maker because the rate of production of impulses is more here.

14. What are the conducting systems of heart?

Ans. Conducting system of heart are formed by the modified cardiac muscle fibers. These fibers are specialized cells that conduct impulses rapidly from Sinoatrial (SA) node to ventricle. Various components of conducting system of heart are **sinoatrial (SA) node, inter nodal fibers, AV node, bundle** of His and **its branches and purkinje** fibers.

15. How rhythmical contraction of heart occurs?

Ans. Heart is consisting of special system that generates rhythmical electrical impulses to cause rhythmical contraction of heart muscle and conducting these impulses rapidly through the heart. Specialized excitatory and conducting system of heart that control cardiac contractions are sinoatrial node (SA) node, intermodal fibers, atrio ventricular node, atrio ventricular (AV) bundle and purkinje fibers. Out of these structures, in **SA node** the normal rhythmical inmpulse is generated. Generated impulse is passed from SA node to AV node through **intermodal fibers**. From **AV node** at atria the impulses is passed to ventricle by **AV bundle**. Gradually AV bundle divides in to two parts as left bundle branches and right bundle branches of **purkinje fibers** which conduct the cardiac impulse to all parts of ventricle.

16. What is anatomy of cardiac muscle?

Ans. Cardiac muscle is striated in the same way as skeletal muscle. Cardiac muscle has myofibrils that contain myocin and actin filaments those are identical to skeletal muscle fibers. These filaments lie side by side and slide along one another during contraction in the same manner as occurs in skeletal muscle. The cell membrane that separate individual cardiac muscle cell from one another is called **intercalated disc**. Cardiac muscle fiber are made up of many individual cells connected in series with one another. The cell membrane of muscle fiber fuse with one another in such a way that they form a permeable communication junction called gap junction which allows free diffusion of ions. So the action potential travel from one cardiac muscle to other passing intercalated disc with negligible hinderance. Therefore cardiac muscle is called **syncytium** of many cells in which cardiac cells are so inter connected that when one of the cell is excited the action potential spreads to all of them. The heart is consisting of two syncytium as **atrial syncytium** and **ventricular syncytium**.

17. What cause the long action potential and plateau in cardiac muscle than skeletal muscle?

Ans This is because of two major differences between membrane properties of cardiac and skeletal muscle. They are as such I) The action potential of skeletal muscle is caused entirely by sudden opening of large number of fast sodium channels. These channels are called fast as it remains open for $10{,}000^{th}$ of a second and then suddenly close but in cardiac muscle the action potential is caused by the opening of two types of channels. They are i) **Fast sodium channel** like in skeletal muscle ii) By **slow calcium channels** called calcium-sodium channels. This slow calcium channel differs from fast sodium channels by slower to open and even remain open for several tenth of a second. During this time a large quantity of both calcium and sodium ions flow through these channels to the interior of the cardiac muscle fiber and this maintains a prolonged period of depolarization causing **plateau** in action potential. II) The second major functional difference between cardiac and skeletal muscle for prolonged action potential and plateau is that immediately after onset of the action potential the permeability of cardiac muscle membrane for potassium ion decreases about 5 fold, the effect that does not occur in the skeletal muscle. This decreased potassium permeability may be caused by the excess calcium influx through the calcium channels. This decreased K^+ permeability greatly decreases the out flux of potassium ions during the action potential plateau and there by prevents early return of action potential to its resting level.

18. What is refractory period of cardiac muscle?

Ans. It is the period during which a normal cardiac impulse can't reexcite an already excited cardiac muscle. Refractory period of ventricle is about 0.25 to 0.3 sec. Refractory period of atrial muscle is much shorter than ventricle which is about 0.15 sec.

19. What is Excitation contraction coupling in heart muscle?

Ans. This term **excitation contraction coupling** refers to the mechanism by which an action potential causes the myofibrils to contract. When action potential passes over cardiac muscle membrane the action potential spreads to the interior of cardiac muscle fiber along the membrane of the **transverse (T) tubules**. This T-tubule action potential in turn acts on membrane of the sarcoplasmic reticulum to release cations into the muscle sarcoplasm. These calcium ions catalyze the chemical reactions that promote sliding of the actin and myosin filaments that causes muscle conduction. This mechanism of excitation contraction coupling is similar to that of skeletal muscle but there is second effect that is different i.e. in addition to the calcium ions released from sarcoplasmic reticulum, large quantity of extra cations also diffuse to sarcoplasm from T-tubules at the time of action potential. Without this extra calcium from T-tubules the contraction of cardiac muscle would be reduced as the sarcoplasmic reticulum of cardiac muscle is less developed than skeletal muscle and does not store enough calcium for full contraction. Skeletal muscle is hardly affected by change in extracellular calcium ion concentration because skeletal muscle contraction is entirely caused by cation released from sarcoplasmic reticulum inside skeletal muscle fiber itself.

20. What is systemic circulation?

Ans. Systemic circulation is otherwise called **greater circulation**. The blood which is pump from left ventricle passes through series of blood vessels of **arterial system** and reaches tissues. The blood vessels of arterial system are aorta, large arteries, small arteries and arterioles. The arterioles branches to capillaries. After exchange of materials at capillaries the blood enters the **venous system** and return to right atrium of heart. Blood vessels of venous system are venules, small veins, large veins and vena cavae. From right atrium blood enters the right ventricle. Thus through systemic circulation the oxygenated blood and the arterial blood is supplied from heart to the tissue and the venous blood returns to the heart from the tissue.

21. What is pulmonary circulation?

Ans. Pulmonary circulation is otherwise called as **lesser circulation**. Blood is pumped from right ventricle to lungs through pulmonary artery. The exchange of gases occurs between blood and alveoli of lungs through pulmonary capillary membrane. The oxygenated blood returns to left atrium through pulmonary veins. Thus left side of heart contain oxygenated blood or arterial blood and right side of heart contains deoxygenated and venous blood.

22. What is volume of blood in different parts of circulation?

Ans. Out of 100% of circulation 84% of entire blood volume of body is in systemic circulation and 16% is in heart and lungs. Out of the 84% of systemic circulation 64% is in vein, 13% is in arteries and 7% is systemic arterioles and capillaries. Heart contain 7% of blood and pulmonary vessels about 9%.

23. What is cardiac cycle?

Ans. Each heart beat consists of two major period called systole and diastole. During systole there is contraction of cardiac muscle and pumping of blood from heart. During diastole there is relaxation of cardiac muscle and filling of blood. Various changes or events occurs in different chambers of heart during each heart beat. These changes are repeated during each heart beat in a cyclic manner. So the changes or events that occur from beginning of one heart beat to beginning of next is called **cardiac cycle**. The phases of cardiac cycle are phase I (atrial systole), phase II (isovolumetric contraction), phase III (maximum ejection and rapid ejection), phase IV (reduced ejection and slow ejection), phase V (protodiastole), phase VI (isovolumetric relaxation period), phase VII (rapid filling), phase VIII (reduced filling (diastasis).

24. What are the heart sounds during cardiac cycle?

Ans. The mechanical activities of heart during each cardiac cycle produces sounds called **heart sound**. Normally the heart sounds are produced due to movement of cardiac muscle, valves of the heart and by passing of blood through chamber of heart. These sounds can be heard by stethoscope and recorded graphically. There are **four heart sounds** produces during each cardiac cycle. The **first and second heart sounds** are prominent and sounds as 'lub' and 'dub'. The 'lub' sound is produced due to closure of AV valve at the beginning of systole and the sound 'dub' is associated with the closure of semilunar valve at the end of systole and onset of diastole. The **third heart sound** is a weak, rumbling sound heard occasionally at the beginning of middle third of diastole during rapid filling period of cardiac cycle. Normally this third heart sound is not audible by stethoscope. It can be heard by microphone. **Fourth heart sound** is produced during atrial systole in some cases and can be recorded graphically by phonocardiogram. This sound is never audible by stethoscope because of its low frequency.

25. What is cardiac murmurs?

Ans. Abnormal heart sounds are called cardiac murmurs or **bruits**. These abnormal heart sounds are produced because of the change in pattern of blood flow. Normally blood flows in a stream through heart or blood vessels but during abnormal condition like vulvular diseases the blood flow becomes turbulent which produces cardiac murmurs. The murmur is produced during vulvular diseases and the other diseases like septal defects and defect in blood vessels. Cardiac murmurs are classified in to three types as systolic murmur, diastolic murmur and continuous murmur.

26. What is patent ductus arteriosus?

Ans. During fetal life lungs are collapsed and the elastic compression of lungs keeps the alveoli collapsed so most of the lungs blood vessels are collapsed. This cause all the pulmonary arterial blood flow through a special artery present in the fetus that connect the pulmonary artery with aorta called **ductus arteriosus**, thus bypassing lungs. As soon as the baby is born and begins to breath the lungs inflate the pulmonary arterial pressure fall and aortic pressure rises because of which forward blood flow through ductus arteriosus ceases suddenly. This new state of backward blood flow through ductus arteriosus does not persists permanently rather this ductus arteriosus is believed to close because back flow of blood has twice as high concentration of oxygen than pulmonary arterial blood that had been flowing in ductus arteriosus during fetal life. This high oxygen in turn cause constriction of muscles in ductus arteriosus wall and finally close it. But in some condition this is not closed and cause the condition called **patent ductus arteriosus.**

27. What is electrocardiogram?

Ans. When cardiac impulse passes through heart there is passes of electrical currents from heart to surrounding tissues. These small currents produced can be recorded by using suitable electrodes by placing them on body on opposite site of heart. Recording of these currents is called **electrocardiogram or ECG**. The instrument used to record this current is called **electrocardiograph** and the technique to record this current is called **electrocardigraphy**. This technique was discovered by Dutch physiologist **Einthoven Willem**. The normal electrocardiogram is composed of P wave, QRS complex and T wave. QRS complex is often composed of three separate waves as 'Q' wave, 'R' wave and 'S' wave but not always. **P wave** is caused by electrical potential generated when the atria depolarize at the beginning of the atrial contraction. **QRS wave** is generated when the ventricle depolarize at the beginning of the ventricular contraction. Both 'P' and "QRS' waves are called as **depolarization wave. T wave** is the potential generated due to repolarization of ventricle.

28. How ECG is recorded?

Ans. The electrical currents generated by the cardiac muscle during each beat of heart change electrical potentials and polarities on the respective sides of the heart in less than 0.01 second. Therefore it is essential that any apparatus for recording electrocardiogram must be capable of responding the changes in potential rapidly. The ECG is recorded by using a set of bipolar and unipolar leads called ECG leads. ECG leads are of two types as **bipolar leads** and **unipolar leads.** In bipolar electrocardiography the electrocardiogram is recorded from two electrodes on different sides of heart i.e on limbs. The bipolar leads are fixed on the limbs. Usually on right arm, left arm and left leg are used. The heart is said to be placed in the center of the imaginary equilateral triangle by connecting root of these three limbs. The triangle is called **Eithoven's triangle**. Unipolar leads are of two types as **unipolar limb leads** and **unipolar chest leads**. In unipolar leads one is active electrode and other one is an indifferent electrode.

29. What is phonocardiogram?

Ans. Normally heart sounds are detected by stethoscope but low frequency heart sounds are detected by phonocardiogram. **Phonocardiogram** is the method to detect low frequency heart sounds graphically by a microphone specially designed to detect these sounds. These low frequency heart sounds are amplified and recorded by a high speed recording apparatus which appears as wave.

30. What is echocardiogram?

Ans. An **echocardiogram** often referred as a sonogram of heart. It is also known as a **cardiac ultrasound**. There are uses of standard ultrasound techniques to image two-dimensional slices of the heart. **Echocardiography** is one of the most widely used diagnostic tests to diagnose cardiovascular diseases. It provide information on size and shape of heart, its pumping capacity, location and extent of damage to its tissues. It is especially useful for assessing diseases of the heart valves and also can detect abnormalities in the pattern of blood flow.

31. What is vectocardiography (VCG)?

Ans. VCG is another means of graphically displaying heart's electrical activity. Vectocardiogram is produced when two simultaneously recorded perpendicular ECG leads are connected to the horizontal and vertical plates of a cathode ray oscilloscope. From ECG only the calculated vector i.e cardiac axis can be determined but by vectocardiogram the instantaneous mean vector can be determined. This instantaneous mean vector can not be determined by ECG.

32. What is cardiac out put?

Ans. It is the quantity of blood pumped to aorta from ventricle/ heart per each minute. This is also defines as the quantity of blood that flow through the circulation. Cardiac out put is the most important factor in cardiovascular system because the rate of blood flow through different parts of the body depends upon the cardiac output.

33. What is stroke volume?

Ans: It is defined as the amount of blood pumped out by each ventricle during each beat. It is of 70 ml (60-80 ml) when heart rate is normal (72/min).

34. What is Minute volume?

Ans. This is the amount of blood pumped out by each ventricle in one minute. This is calculated by multiplying stroke volume with heart rate. Normal value of minute volume is 5L/ ventricle/ minute.

35. What is cardiac index?

Ans. It is the cardiac output per square meter of body surface area. It is defined as the amount of blood pumped out of ventricle per minute per square meter of the body surface area. Normal cardiac index of an adult is $3L/min/m^2$ of body surface area. Fever, anemia, hyperthyroidism normally increases cardiac output where as hypothyroidism, atrial fibrillation, myocardial degeneration, congestive cardiac failure, shock and hemorrhage decreases cardiac output.

36. What is Coronary circulation?

Ans. Blood circulation to heart is called coronary circulation. Blood supply to heart muscle is by two coronary arteries i.e right and left coronary arteries which are the first branches of aorta. Main coronary arteries lies on the surface of heart and smaller arteries then penetrate from the surface into cardiac muscle mass. Left coronary artery supply anterior and left lateral portion of left ventricle where as right coronary artery supplies most of the right ventricle as well as posterior part of the left ventricle. Coronary arteries divide and subdivide into smaller branches which run all along the surface of the heart. The smaller branches are called **epicardial arteries** and give rise to further smaller branches called **final arteries** or **intramural vessels.** The final arteries run at right angle through the heart muscle near the inner aspect of wall of heart. The venous drainage or flow from the heart muscle is by three types of vessels as **coronary sinus, anterior coronary veins** and **thebesian veins.**

37. What is myocardial infarction?

Ans. Because of an acute coronary occlusion if a large part of myocardium is involved, that leads to ischemia. The area of myocardium that has either zero blood flow or absolutely less flow there is ischemia so cardiac muscle function can not be sustained and that leads to necrosis (death of part of myocardium). This condition is called **myocardial infarction**. Myocardial infarction cause death due to decrease in cardiac out put, pulmonary edema, ventricular fibrillation and rupture of heart.

38. What is myocardial stunning?

Ans. Due to infarcted area the blood vessels become dilated and there will be over filled of stagnant blood and gradually this stagnant blood become deoxygenated and give bluish brown colour to the area. Finally in later stage the vessel wall become highly permeable and leak fluid so the local tissue become edematous and cardiac muscle cells begin to swell because of diminized cellular metabolism. Substantial reduced in coronary blood flow cause ischemia followed by necrosis. This ischemia or necrosis produce mechanical disturbances or dysfunction of heart. is called **myocardial stunning**.

39. What is angina pectoris?

Ans. Ischemic cardiac muscle often cause pain sensation in heart and some times severe pain. It is believed that ischemia cause muscle to release acidic substances like lactic acid and other pain promoting products such as histamine, kinis or cellular proteolytic enzymes. High concentration of these products stimulate nerve endings in cardiac muscle that send pain impulse through sensory afferent nerve fiber. This pain due to myocardial ischemia is called **angina pectoris or cardiac pain**. This cardiac pain is also called as referred pain as it is felt over the body away from heart. This pain is also spread to left arm, left shoulder, neck as well as side of the face. The reason for this distribution of pain is that the heart originates during embryonic life in the neck as do the arms. Therefore both the heart and these surface area of the body receives pain nerve fibers from same spinal cord segments.

40. How pumping of heart is regulated?

Ans. During rest the heart pumps 4-6L of blood in each minute. During severe exercise the heart pumps 4-7 times more than rest blood. So the means by which blood is pumped by the heart is regulated are **intrinsic cardiac regulation of pumping** in response to changes in volume of blood flowing in to heart and control of heart rate and strength of heart pumping by autonomic nervous system called **extrinsic regulation of pumping. By intrinsic regulation of heart pumping** the amount of blood pumped by heart in each minute is determined almost entirely by the rate of blood flow into heart from the veins called venous return. The intrinsic ability of heart to adapt to increasing volumes of inflowing blood is called **Frank starling mechanism** of the heart. The pumping effectiveness of heart is also controlled by autonomic nervous system through sympathetic and parasympathetic nerves. This regulation of heart pumping is called **extrinsic regulation of heart pumping.** Sympathetic stimulation increases heart rate as well as force of contraction there by increasing the volume of blood pumped and increasing the ejection pressure. Strong parasympathetic (vagal) nerve stimulation can stop heart beat for a few seconds but then the heart usually escapes and bet at rate of 20-40 beats per minute about 40% of normal. Strong vagal stimulation decrease the strength of heart contraction by 20-30%.

41. What is the effect of electrolytes on heart function?

Ans. The distribution of electrolytes in extra cellular fluid and intra cellular fluid are responsible for the electrical activity of the tissues including myocardium. Thus any change in the concentration of any of the electrolytes alters the electrical activity of the cardiac muscle. It has already been discussed that sodium and potassium ions have marked effect on membrane potential and action potential and calcium ion have an important role in activating muscle contraction. Therefore it is to be expected that concentration of these ions have important effect on cardiac pumping.

42. What is the effect of temperature on heart function?

Ans. Increase in temperature of body as in fever cause greatly increase in heart rate where as decrease in temperature cause decrease in heart rate. This effect may be concluded that heat causes increased permeability of the cardiac muscle membrane to the controlling ions. Contractile strength of the heart often is enhanced temporarily by moderate increase in temperature but prolonged elevation of temperature exhaust the metabolic system of heart and eventually cause weakness. Therefore optimal function of the heart depends greatly on proper control of body temperature.

43. What is Hemodynamics?

Ans. Dynamics means study of motion and **hemodynamics** means the study of movement of blood through circulatory system. The major function of cardiovascular system is to pump the blood and to circulate it through different parts of the body and to transport nutrients to body tissue and to transport waste product away from the body. It is essential to maintain pressure and other physical factors within blood vessels so that the volume of blood supplied to different parts of the body is adequate.

44. What are different types of blood flow in body?

Ans. Flow of blood or fluid is of two types as

i) Stream line or laminar flow

It is flow of blood at a steady rate through blood vessel. Stream line flow is silent flow. This type of flow does not produce sound within blood vessel.

ii) Turbulent flow

When velocity of blood flow increases at critical level the flow become turbulent and creates sound. In this flow, blood flow in all directions in the vessel and continually mixing within vessel.

45. What is Blood pressure?

Ans. Generally blood pressure refers to **arterial** blood pressure. It is the pressure exerted by blood on the wall of arteries. This pressure is exerted when blood flows through arteries. Blood pressure is expressed in four different terms as i) **systolic pressure:** it is the maximum pressure exerted in the arteries during systole of heart, ii) **diastolic pressure:** it is the minimum pressure in the arteries during diastole of heart, iii) **pulse pressure:** this is the difference between systolic and diastolic pressure and iv) **mean arterial blood pressure:** this is the average pressure existing in the arteries. This is not the arithmetic mean of systolic and diastolic pressures. This is the diastolic pressure plus $1/3^{rd}$ of pulse pressure.

46. What are the Factors to maintain blood pressure?

Ans. There are factors necessary to maintain normal blood pressure are called local factors. These factors are **central factors** and **peripheral factors**. Central factors are cardiac out put and heart rate. Peripheral factors are peripheral resistance, blood volume, venous return, elasticity of blood vessel, velocity of blood flow, diameter of blood vessels, and viscosity of blood.

47. How arterial blood pressure is regulated?

Ans. Body has four regulatory mechanism to regulate blood pressure they are i) Nervous mechanism or short term regulatory mechanism, ii) Renal mechanism or long term regulatory mechanism, iii) Hormonal mechanism and iv) Local mechanism.

48. What is short term regulatory mechanism to regulate blood pressure?

Ans. Short term regulatory mechanism to regulate blood pressure is by nervous mechanism which constitute vasomotor system. Regulation of blood pressure by nervous system is rapid among all the mechanism. It operates only for a short period so called short term regulation. This vasomotor system include components like **vasomotor center, vasoconstrictor fiber and vasodilator fiber.** Vasomotor center to control blood pressure are located in medulla oblongata and pons. Vasoconstrictor fibers belongs to sympathetic division autonomic nervous system. These fibers cause vasoconstriction by release of neurotransmitter called noradrenalin which acts through β-receptor of smooth muscle fiber of blood vessels. Vasodilator fiber cause dilation of the blood vessel and are of three types as **parasympathetic vasodilator fiber, sympathetic vasodilator fiber** and **antidromic vasodilator fiber**.

49. What is antidromic vasodilator fiber?

Ans. Impulse produce by cutaneous receptor pass through sensory nerve fibers but some impulse pass through other branches of axon and reach blood vessels. These impulse now dilate blood vessels. This is called **antidromic axon reflex** and the nerve fiber involves are called antidromic vasodilator fiber.

50. What is vasovagal syncope?

Ans. A typical vasodilatory reaction is seen in people who experience intense emotional disturbances that cause fainting. In this case the muscle vasodilator system becomes activated and at the same time vagal cardio inhibitory center transmits strong signal to heart which markedly slow down the heart rate. So the arterial pressure falls instantly which reduces blood flow to the brain and cause the person to lose consciousness. This effect is called **vasovagal syncope**.

51. How vasomotor center regulate blood pressure?

Ans. Vasomotor center regulates arterial blood pressure by causing vasoconstriction or vasodilation. However its action depends upon the impulse receives from other structures such as **baroreceptors, chemoreceptors, higher center** and **respiratory center**. Baroreceptors and chemoreceptors play major role in the short term regulation of blood pressure.

52. What is the action of baroreceptor to control blood pressure?

Ans. Baroreceptors are called **pressoreceptors**. These are the receptors which give response to change in blood pressure. Baroreceptors are present in carotid sinus and aorta. When arterial blood pressure rises rapidly the baroreceptors are activated then, which in turn send stimulatory impulse to nucleus of tractus solitaries. Now nucleus of tractus solitaries acts on both vasoconstrictor area and vasodilator area of vasomotor center. It inhibits vasoconstrictor area and excites vasodilator area. The fall of arterial blood pressure decrease pressure in carotid sinus that cause inactivation of baroreceptors and cause rise in blood pressure.

53. What is the action of chemoreceptor to control blood pressure?

Ans. **Chemoreceptors** are the receptors giving response to change in chemical constituents of blood. Peripheral chemoreceptors influence vasomotor center which are situated in the carotid body and aortic body. Chemoreceptors are sensitive to lack of oxygen, excess of carbon dioxide and hydrogen ion concentration in blood. Whenever blood pressure decreases the blood flow decreases resulting decrease in oxygen content and excess of carbon dioxide and hydrogen ion concentration. These factors stimulate chemoreceptors which send impulse to excite vasoconstrictor center because of which blood pressure increases and blood flow increases.

54. How higher centers control blood pressure?

Ans. The vasomotor center is also controlled by impulse from two higher centers of brain such as cerebral cortex and hypothalamus. **Cerebral cortex** is concerned with emotional reactions. During emotional condition this area sends impulse to vasomotor center so that vasomotor center is activated which cause increase in blood pressure. Stimulation of anterior hypothalamus cause vasodilation and decrease in blood pressure. Stimulation of posterior hypothalamus cause vasoconstriction and increase in blood pressure.

55. How respiratory center acts to control blood pressure?

Ans. During expiration arterial blood pressure increases slightly and it decreases during later part of expiration and during inspiration. This is because of two factors ad i) radiation of impulse from respiratory center towards vasomotor center at different phases of respiratory cycle. ii) Pressure changes in thoracic cavity leads to alteration of venous return and cardiac output.

56. What is renal mechanism or long term regulatory mechanism to regulate blood pressure?

Ans. Kidney plays an important role in long term regulation of blood pressure. Renin is a small enzyme which is a protein in nature synthesized and stored in an inactive form called prorenin in the juxta glomerular (JG) cells of kidney. When the arterial pressure falls too low intrinsic reactions in the kidney cause many of the prorenin molecules in the JG cells to split and release rennin. Most of the rennin enters the renal blood and then passes out of the kidneys and circulate throughout the body. Renin acts enzymatically on another plasma protein, a globulin called angiotensinogen (produced in liver) and concert it to **angiotensin I** a 10 amino acid peptide. Within few seconds after formation of angiotensin I it converted to **angiotensin II** a 8 amino acid peptide by converting enzyme secreted from endothelium of lungs. Angiotensin II is an extremely powerful **vasoconstrictor**. Vasoconstriction occurs intensively in arterioles and much less in veins. Constriction of arterioles increases peripheral resistance thereby raising arterial pressure. Mild constriction of the veins promote increase in venous return of blood to the heart thereby helping to increase systemic blood pressure also. Angiotensin II also activate **aldosterone** secretion from adrenal cortex. Aldosterone stimulate sodium reabsorption in the cortical and medulary collecting ducts which increase in ECF volume that finally leads to increase in arterial blood pressure.

57. What are the hormones responsible to regulate blood pressure?

Ans. Hormones which are responsible to increase blood pressure are adrenaline, nor adrenaline, thyroxine, aldosterone, vasopressin, angiotensin, serotonin etc but the hormones which are responsible to decrease blood pressure are vasoactive intestinal polypeptide (VIP), bradykinin, prostaglandin, histamine, acetyle choline, atrial natriuretic peptide etc.

58. What are the local mechanisms to regulate blood pressure?

Ans. The local substances that regulate the blood pressure by causing vasoconstriction and vasodilation. Local vasoconstrictor substances secreted from endothelial cells of blood vessels are **endothelins (ET)**. These endothelins are ET1, ET2 and ET3. These endothelins are produced because of stretching of blood vessels. These endothelins acts by activating phospholipase which in turn activate prostacyclin and thromboxane A2. These two substances cause constriction of blood vessels and increase blood pressure. Local vasodilators are of two types as vasodilator of metabolic origin and vasodilator of endothelial origin. Vasodilator of metabolic origin are carbon dioxide, lactate, hydrogen ions and adenosine where as vasodilators of endothelial origin is nitric oxide (NO). This NO is a vasodilator so cause decrease in blood pressure.

59. What is venous pressure?

Ans. The pressure exerted by blood in the vein is called as venous pressure. This pressure is not same in all veins. Venous pressure is less in the part of the body which are above the level of heart and it is less in the part of the body which are below the level of heart. **Venous pressure is greater in peripheral veins than central veins.** Blood from all the systemic veins flows into the right atrium of the heart therefore the pressure in the right atrium is called **central venous pressure**. Right atrial pressure is regulated by a balance between i) ability of heart to pump blood out of the right atrium and ventricle and ii) tendency for blood to flow from peripheral veins into right atrium.

60. What is function of capillaries?

Ans. Important function of capillary is to exchange of substance between blood and tissue. Oxygen, nutrients, water and other essential substances enter the tissue from capillary blood and carbon dioxide, metabolites and other unwanted substances are removed from the tissue by capillary blood. Most important means by which substances are transferred between plasma and interstitial fluid is **diffusion.** The other means by which exchange of materials occurs across the capillary endothelium are **filtration** and **pinocytosis**.

61. How fetal circulation is different from that of adult?

Ans. Fetal circulation is different from that of adult. This is due to presence of placenta which is responsible for exchange of gases between fetal blood and mother's blood because fetal lungs are non functional. Fetus is connected with mother through placenta. Fetal blood passes to placenta through umbilical vessels and maternal blood runs through uterine vessels. These two blood vessels lie in close proximity in placenta through which the exchange of substance takes place between mother's blood and fetal blood. Fetal lungs are non functional, so the blood bypass them. From placenta the **umbilical vein** collects blood (which is rich in oxygen) and nutrients and supply to fetal body. About half of the blood from umbilical vein is supplied to the liver of fetus. However rest half of the blood is diverted from umbilical vein into inferior vena cavae through **ductus venosus** which bypass liver. The ductus venosus travels a short distance and joins with inferior vena cavae, there the oxygenated blood from placenta is mixed with deoxygenated blood from lower parts of body. Both oxygenated and deoxygenated blood mixture enters right atrium via inferior vena cavae. From right atrium large portion of blood pass to left atrium through an opening called **foramen ovale**. But in adult, blood from right atrium goes to right ventricle then through pulmonary artery it goes to lungs. In fetus lungs are non functional so the blood bypass them. A small valve called **septum primum** is located on the left side of the atrial septum overlies foramen ovale and helps to prevent blood from moving in reverse direction. The rest of the fetal blood enter right atrium including large portion of deoxygenated blood from upper part of the body enters right atrium through superior vena cavae. Both the blood from right atrium enters right ventricle. From right ventricle blood is pumped to **pulmonary artery**. From pulmonary artery blood enters systemic aorta through **ductus arteriosus or ductus botalli** (as lungs in fetus is collapsed). From this aorta some of blood is supplied to various parts of the body and rest passes into **umbilical artery** which is branched from **internal iliac artery** and leads to placenta.

62. What is lymphatic system?

Ans. Lymphatic system represents an accessory route through which fluid can flow from interstitial space into blood. Lymphatic system carries proteins and large particles from tissue space to blood stream. The steady state of tissue space depends upon the passage of materials in and out of the blood capillaries and passage of materials into lymph system and then back to the blood stream. The excess of capillary filtration over reabsorption is balanced by lymph flow. Lymphatic system helps to maintain the fluid balance between blood vessel and tissue.

63. What are the functions of lymph?

Ans. There are many function of lymph as

i) Important function of lymph is to return the proteins from tissue space to blood.

ii) Lymph flow plays an important role in redistribute of fluid in the body.

iii) Through lymph, bacteria, toxins and other foreign bodies are removed from tissue.

iv) Lymph flow is responsible for maintenance of structural and functional integrity of tissue.

v) Lymph flow serves as an important route for intestinal fat absorption.

vi) Lymph also plays an important role in immunity by transporting lymphocytes.

64. What is Shock and its cause?

Ans. **Circulatory shock**, commonly known as **shock** is a serious life threatening condition due to an inadequate perfusion (blood flow) of tissues which become insufficient to meet cellular metabolic needs. Because of shock too little blood (little oxygen and nutrients) is supplied to the tissues that cause damage to tissue. Shock is usually results from inadequate cardiac out put. Therefore any condition that reduces the cardiac out put far below normal will likely lead to circulatory shock. There are two factors that severely reduce cardiac out put, they are i) cardiac abnormalities that decrease the ability of heart to pump blood ii) factors that decreases venous return also decreases cardiac output. Sometimes shock also results without diminized cardiac output. This condition can result from i) excessive metabolism of body so that even a normal cardiac output is inadequate, ii) abnormal tissue perfusion pattern so that most of the cardiac output is passing through blood vessels besides those that supply the local tissue with nutrition.

65. What are the stages of shock?

Ans. On the basis of degree of severity shock is divided in to three major stages as

i) **Non progressive stage or compensated stage**

In this stage normal circulatory compensatory mechanism cause full recovery of shock without help of outside therapy.

ii) **Progressive stage**

This stage is otherwise called as **decompensating** stage. In this stage shock become steadily worse and compensatory mechanisms begin to fail until death.

iii) **Irreversible stage**

This stage is otherwise called as **refractory** stage. In this stage shock has progressed to such an extent that all forms of known therapy becomes inadequate to save person's life.

Choose the Best Answer

1. **Death of an area of tissue due to interrupted blood supply is called**
   a) Ischemia
   b) Angina pectoris
   c) Thrombosis
   d) Infarction

2. **Cardio acceleratory center is located in the**
   a) Cerebrum
   b) Pons
   c) Medulla
   d) Spinal cord

3. **Which of the following statements about arteries is incorrect**
   a) All arteries carry oxygenated blood from the heart
   b) They do not contain valves as do veins
   c) All arteries carry blood away from the heart
   d) They have large amounts of elastic tissue

4. **Which of the following does not contribute to the return of blood to the heart**
   a) Valves associated with veins
   b) Contractions of skeletal muscle
   c) Breathing
   d) Fact that veins are stronger than arteries

5. **Main determinant of blood pressure is**
   a) Peripheral resistance
   b) Blood volume
   c) Elasticity of arteries
   d) Cardiac output

6 **Blood flows because of**
   a) Beating of the heart
   b) Establishment of a pressure gradient
   c) Establishment of a concentration gradient
   d) Elasticity of the arteries

7. **Approximately, how much blood flows directly through the atria into the ventricles even before the atria contract**
   a) 20% - 30%
   b) 40% - 50%
   c) 70% - 80%
   d) 90%-100%

8. When the pressure in the left ventricle exceeds than in the aorta, then

a) Tripcuspid valve open
b) Blood flows into the ventricles
c) P-wave of the ECG begin
d) Semilunar valve open

9. Aspirin reduce the risk of heart disease because

a) It is a powerful vasodilator
b) It blocks pain receptors in heart tissue
c) It stops ventricular fibrillation
d) It prevents platelet clumping

10. Hematocrit measures percentage of

a) White blood cells b) Plasma
c) Platelets d) Red blood cells

11. Granulocytes are formed in

a) Kidney b) Liver
c) Bone marrow d) Small intenstine

12. Blood component that plays major role in maintaining the osmotic pressure of blood is

a) Albumin b) Carbon dioxide
c) White blood cells d) Fibrinogen

13. Increase in number of RBC in blood is called

a) Anemia b) Polycythemia
c) Leucopenia d) Thrombocytopenia

14. Most of the carbon dioxide produced by tissues is transported to the lungs as

a) Small gas bubbles in the plasma
b) Gas bound to hemoglobin in the red blood cells
c) Bicarbonate ions in the plasma
d) Gas bound to white blood cells and albumin

15. To prevent blood loss after a tissue injury, blood vessels first

a) Form a platelet plug
b) Form a clot
c) Initiate the coagulation cascade
d) Constrict and form barriers

16. Which of the following cells is most abundant in human blood

a) Neutrophils b) Basophils
c) Eosinophils d) Monocytes

17. A bag of donated blood does not clot because

a) There is not enough oxygen
b) It can not dry out
c) It is kept refrigerated
d) There is no free calcium

18. Which one conducts electricity like nerves

a) Epicardium b) Pericardium
c) Myocardium d) Subvalaular Apparatus

19. Who carries most blood at any given time in body

a) Veins b) Capillary Beds
c) Aorta d) Vena Cava

20. Which of the following contract together to pump blood

a) Right atrium with the right ventricle and left atrium with the left ventricle
b) Right atrium with left atrium and right ventricles with left ventricle
c) Tricuspid valve and mitral valve
d) Aorta and pulmonary artery

21. Pacemaker of the heart is

a) AV node b) Purkinje fibers
c) AV Bundle d) SA node

22. In ECG which letter shows the depolarization from the AV node down to the AV bundle

a) S b) P
c) T d) Q

23. T wave in an ECG shows

a) Resting potential
b) Atrial depolarization
c) SA node excitation
d) Ventricle repolarization

24. Blood pressure is the measure of

a) Pressure exerted by the blood on the walls of the blood vessels
b) Pressure exerted by the blood on the arteries
c) Pressure exerted by the blood on the veins
d) Pressure exerted by the blood on the aorta

25. Systolic Pressure is

a) An average of 120 mm Hg
b) Lowers steadily during ventricle systole
c) The highest when blood is being pumped out of the left ventricle into the aorta
d) An average of 80 mm Hg
e) Both a and c

26. Heart has how many chambers

a) One
b) Two
c) Three
d) Four

27. Plasma is

a) Blood that has no red blood cells
b) Liquid portion of blood including clotting factors
c) Liquid portion of blood after it has clotted
d) Proteins of blood

28. Excessive destruction of erythrocytes can result in

a) Thalassemia
b) Aplastic anemia
c) Pericious anemia
d) Hemolytic anemia

29. Hematocrit value of 80 is termed as

a) Polycythemia
b) Anemia
c) Thrombocytopenia
d) Leukemia

30. During hemoglobin recycling, heme is converted to

a) Bilirubin
b) Biliverdin
c) Urobilin
d) Urobilinogen

31. Heme portion of hemoglobin is

a) Converted into stercobilin in the large intestine
b) Converted into urobilin in the kidney
c) Excreted from the body
d) All of the above

32. Fe^{3+} portion of hemaglobin is

a) Converted into transferrin in the large intestine
b) Converted into ferritin in the kidney
c) Excreted from the body
d) None of the above

33. Increase in neutrophil count is associated with

a) Bacterial infection
b) Neutropenia
c) Allergic reactions
d) Parasitic infections

34. Cells which are important phagocytes and eventually become macrophage

a) Neutrophils
b) Basophils
c) Monocytes
d) Lymphocytes

35. Hypoxia induces kidneys to produce

a) Platelets
b) Intrinsic factor
c) Urobilin
d) Erythropoetin

36. First phase of hemostasis is

a) Separation of globin and heme
b) Activation of prothrombinase
c) Platelet aggregation
d) Vascular spasm

37. Which of the following activates platelets during hemostasis

a) Eosinophil degranulation
b) Exposed collagen or endothelial basement membrane
c) Fibrin thread formation
d) Thromboplastin

38. Phase of coagulation that begins with exposed endothelial collagen is

a) Extrinsic pathway b) Intrinsic pathway
c) Common pathway d) Fibrin stabilization

39. Which clotting factor is an important link between the intrinsic and extrinsic pathways and is deficient in hemophilia B

a) Factor IX b) Factor XII
c) Factor VIII d) Fibrinogen

40. Which clotting factor plays an important role in activating two positive feedback loops to accelerate coagulation

a) Thrombin b) Fibrin
c) Calcium d) Prothrombinase

41. An individual with type B+ blood has which of the following antibodies in their blood

a) Anti-A and anti-O b) Anti-B
c) Anti-Rh d) Anti-A

42. The space in the middle of the thoracic cavity where the heart resides is the

a) Pericardial cavity b) Pericardium
c) Pleural cavity d) Mediastinum

43. Foramen ovale in the fetal heart is located in

a) Right atrium b) Left atrium
c) Interventricular septum d) Interatrial septum

44. Which blood vessel does not bring blood directly to the heart

a) Cardiac vein b) Coronary sinus
c) Inferior vena cava d) Superior vena cava

45. If communication between the SA node and the AV node becomes blocked which is most certainly affected

a) Ventricles will contract at a slower rat
b) After load will increase
c) Atria will contract at a slower rate
d) Stroke volume will increase

46. If there is a blockage between the AV node and AV bundle, the appearance of the ECG will

a) P-R interval would be smaller
b) QRS interval would be longer
c) There would be more P waves than QRS complexes
d) There would be more QRS complexes than P waves

47. Neutrophills serve as

a) Mapping up
b) Histiocytes
c) Macrophages
d) Microphages

48. A valve damaged by rheumatic fever fails to open completely is called

a) Stenosis
b) Heart block
c) Ischemia
d) Fibrillation

49. Cation necessary for coagulation of blood is

a) Na
b) K
c) Ca
d) Cl

50. Blood returning from the lungs enters the heart through

a) Pulmonary semilunar valve
b) Mitral valve
c) Right ventricle
d) Left atrium

51. According to Starling's Law of the heart, cardiac output is directly related to

a) Size of the ventricles
b) Heart rate
c) Amount of blood returning to heart
d) End-systolic volume

52. T wave on an ECG represents

a) Ventricular depolarization
b) Ventricular repolarization
c) Atrial depolarization
d) Atrial repolarization

53. Cardiac output is equal to

a) Diastolic BP + 1/3 (systolic BP- diastolic BP)
b) HR x SV
c) EDV-ESV
d) EDV-SV x HR

54. During ventricular systole

a) Atria are contracting
b) AV valves are closed
c) Pressure inside ventricles is less than atria
d) Mitral valve is closed

55. Veins exhibit different character when compared to arteries is

a) Veinsare thinner walled
b) Veins have more smooth muscle in tunica Media
c) Veins carry faster moving blood
d) Veins have thicker endothelium

56. The blood vessels that play the most important role in the regulation of blood flow to a tissue and blood pressure are the

a) Arterioles b) Capillaries
c) Venules d) Arteries

57. As blood travels from the aorta to capillaries

a) Pressure increases b) Viscosity increases
c) Resistance increases d) Velocity increases

58. Internal carotids and basilar artery are interconnected by an anastomosis call

a) Brachiocephalic trunk b) Common carotid artery
c) Coronary sinus d) Circle of Willis

59. Hematology is the study of

a) Bone b) Blood
c) Haemoglobin d) Cartilage

60. The difference between the systolic and diastolic pressures is called

a) Mean arterial blood pressure
b) Blood pressure
c) Pulse pressure
d) End-ventricular pressure

61. Which of the following is not a risk factor for developing atherosclerosis

a) High dietary fat intake
b) Diabetes
c) Smoking
d) High HDL level

62. Which statement regarding blood cells is correct

a) All blood cells originate in red bone marrow
b) Red bone marrow is the primary source of all blood cells except mast cells and macrophage
c) Most types of leukocytes appear in equal amounts in the blood
d) Erythrocytes are produced in red marrow while leukocytes are produced primarily in lymph nodes

63. Organs where activation of T and B cells occur

a) Bone marrow
b) Thymus
c) Lymph nodes
d) All of the above

64. Lymph is returned to general circulation by

a) Superior vena cava
b) Azygos and hemiazygos veins
c) Cisterna chili
d) Subclavian veins

65. Which are most numerous in Cattle blood

a) Lymphocytes
b) Neutrophils
c) Monocytes
d) Eosinophils

66. All the cell granules are absent in

a) Human monocyte
b) WBC
c) Embroy cell
d) Mammalian RBC

67. Carbonic anhydrase is present high concentration in

a) Plasma
b) RBC
c) WBC
d) Nephron

68. Blood protein involved in blood coagulation is

a) Thrombin
b) Fibrinogen
c) Prothrombin
d) Fibrinoprotein

69. Number of RBCs (in million) per mm^3 of human blood is

a) 5.5
b) 7
c) 9
d) 11

70. The liquid left in the blood after removal of all blood cells is called

a) Serum b) Plasma
c) Lymph d) All

71. Main plasma protein is

a) Albumin b) Globulin
c) Fibrinogen d) None

72. All plasma proteins except globulin are formed in

a) Lymphoid organ b) Spleen
c) Bone marrow d) Liver

73. RBC of camel is

a) Circular and nucleated b) Oval and nucleated
c) Oval and non-cleated d) Circular non-nucleated

74. Globin protein is attached to heam by

a) Co-ordinated blood b) Covalent bond
c) Ionic bond d) Hydrogen bond

75. One gram of hemoglobin binds to how much of oxygen

a) 19.6ml b) 1.34ml
c) 4ml d) 20ml

76. Heparin in blood is liberated from

a) Mast cell b) Basophill
c) Both d) None

77. Non-nucleated cell in mammalian blood is

a) RBC b) Leucocyte
c) Muscle cell d) Nerve cell

78. At high altitude the RBCs in human blood

a) Increase in size b) Increase in number
c) Decrease in size d) Decrease in number

79. Proteolytic enzyme that induces lysis of fibrin during fibrinolysis is

a) Fibrin b) Plasmin
c) Thrombin d) Platelet factor VIII

80. Which is a natural anticoagulant

a) Heparin b) Hirudin
c) EDTA d) a & b

81. Reticulocytes are

a) Immatured RBC b) WBC
c) Platelets d) Lymphocytes

82. The ratio of RBC to WBC in cattle blood is

a) 600:1 b) 800:1
c) 1000:1 d) 1300:1

83. The ratio of RBC to WBC in dog blood is

a) 400:1 b) 800:1
c) 1000:1 d) 1300:1

84. Life span (in days) of mammalian RBC is

a) 40 b) 60
c) 120 d) 160

85. One hemoglobin carry how many oxygen atoms

a) 2 b) 4
c) 6 d) 8

86. Blood group where antigen is absent

a) A b) B
c) AB d) O

87. Blood group where antibody is absent

a) A b) B
c) AB d) O

88. Chemical nature of antibody is

a) Protein b) Carbohydrate
c) Fat d) Enzyme

89. Iron present in hemoglobin is

a) Fe+2 form b) Fe+3 form
c) Fe+ form d) All correct

90. Process by which WBC comes out of cell is

a) Excocytosis b) Endocytosis
c) Diapedesis d) None

91. Decrease in Number of WBC is

a) Leucopenia b) Leucocytosis
c) Leukemia d) Polycythemia

92. Antiserum contains

a) Antigens b) Leucocytes
c) Antibodies d) None

93. Blood platelets are the source of

a) Fibrinogen b) Ca+2
c) Thromboplastin d) Hemoglobin

94. Increase in number of RBC in blood is called

a) Polycythemia b) Anemia
c) Leucopenia d) Thrombocytopenia

Answers

1. d	2. c	3. a	4. d	5. a	6. b	7. c	8. d	9. e	10.d
11. c	12. a	13. b	14. c	15. d	16. a	17. d	18. c	19. a	20b
21. d	22. d	23. d	24. a	25. e	26. d	27. b	28. d	29. a	30. a
31. d	32. d	33. a	34. c	35. d	36. d	37. b	38. b	39. a	40. a
41. d	42. d	43. d	44. a	45. a	46. c	47. d	48. a	49. c	50. d
51. c	52. b	53. b	54. b	55. a	56. a	57. c	58. d	59. b	60. c
61. d	62. a	63. c	64. d	65. a	66. d	67. b	68. b	69. a	70. b
71. a	72. d	73. c	74. a	75. b	76. c	77. a	78. b	79. b	80. d
81. a	82. b	83. a	84. c	85. c	86. d	87. c	88. a	89. a	90. c
91. a	92. c	93. c	94. a						

□□□

CHAPTER-3

Digestive System

Depending on food habits **carnivores** have short and simple digestive tract and **herbivores** have large and complex digestive tract. *Pre gastric* fermenting animals are sheep, goat and cattle where fermentation takes place at proximal to gastric digestion. **Post gastric** fermenting animal is horse where fermentation takes place at distal part of digestive tract. Methods of prehension varies in animals but lip, teeth and tongue are the principal organs of prehension. **Dog** and **cat** use fore limb to hold food but pass in to mouth by head and jaw. **Horse** use mobile lips and incisor teeth for prehension, in **cattle** and **sheep** tongue is the principal prehensile organ but food get in by incisor teeth and dental pad. Lower lip is the prehensile organ of *pig*. In simple stomach **cardiac** region is closest to oesophagus that contain cardiac glands which secretes mucous but not enzymes. The body of the stomach is called **fundic** region and contain fundic or gastric glands which are composed of i) **body chief cells** that secretes pepsinogen and gastric enzymes. These chief cells contain small granules called **zymogen granules** substances from which gastric enzymes are derived ii) *neck* **chief cells** that secretes mucous and iii) **parietal cells** that secretes hydrochloric acid and intrinsic factors. Main function of stomach is mixing and storage of ingested food and initiation of protein and fat digestion.

Alimentary canal of ruminant is much more complex than that of non-ruminant because of four parts of stomach in ruminant as i) rumen or paunch ii) reticulum or honey comb iii) omasum or many plies iv) abomesum or true stomach. **Hydrolysis** is the basic process in digestion. **Fat** digestion and absorption occurs exclusively in the small intestine, where as digestion and absorption of **carbohydrate** and **protein** occurs in both small and large intestine. Monogastric digestion is mainly by enzymes but polygastric digestion is by microbial fermentation. Microbes responsible for fermentation are consists mainly of bacteria, fungi and protozoa. The fermentation end products are volatile fatty acids mainly acetic acid, propionic acid and butyric acid with gases like carbon dioxide and methane. Anatomy of avian alimentary canal differs most notably from that of mammal in the mouth area, presence of crop in oesophagus and presence of muscular stomach (gizzard or ventriculus). There are no soft palate in poultry. There is no teeth in poultry but salivary glands and taste buds are present. During digestion of food particles, the large particles from stomach goes to distal part of intestine by the motility pattern is called **migrating myoelectric complexes (MMC)**. This MMC is divided into three phases as **Phase I:** This is a quiescent period during which slow waves are present but no action potential is generated. **Phase II***:* There is presence of intermittent action potential. **Phase III***:* There is intense burst of spike accompanying each slow waves that results in strong gastric contraction.

Gastrointestinal tract is the largest endocrine organ of the body. Here there is secretion of peptide hormones and amines that are released from the cells distributed throughout gastric, intestinal and pancreatic tissue on appropriate simulation. There are three gastrointestinal hormones named **gastrin, secretin and cholecystokinin (CCK). Secretin, gastric inhibitory polypeptide** and **enteroglucagon** are three structurally homologous group which inhibit gastric acid secretion, stimulate pancreatic fluid and bicarbonate secretion, stimulate intestinal secretion, stimulate billiary fluid secretion and alter insulin release. There are three types of salivary glands which are paired are present in the mucous membrane of mouth. They are i) **Parotid** ii) **Sub maxillary (mandibular)** iii) **Sub lingual**. Out of these salivary glands parotid gland produce majority (half) of saliva.

The secretion of submaxillary and parotid glands of non ruminants is **hypotonic** but of ruminants is **isotonic**. So ruminant saliva is highly buffered. Saliva contain chief digestive enzyme **amylase** but this enzyme is absent in carnivores and ruminants. Salivary secretion is controlled by both sympathetic and parasympathetic stimulation. The main substances in body that stimulate parietal cells to secrete hydro chloric acid are acetyl choline, gastrin and histamine. There are three phases of gastric acid secretion as :

i) **Cephalic phase:** This phase of stimulation is result of central stimulation by sigh, smell or taste of food, chewing or swallowing. This response is mediated entirely by vagus nerve.

ii) **Gastric phase:** This phase of secretion occurs as a result of presence of food in stomach. This phase includes both vagal and local neural reflexes. Gastrin and Acetyl choline in this phase also stimulate the parietal cells to secrete hydro chloric acid.

iii) **Intestinal Phase:** This phase begins when food enters the duodenum. One or more hormones released from the duodenal mucosa stimulate gastric secretion. Gastrin and cholecystokinin (CCK) plays important role in this phase.

Food may be carbohydrate, protein or fat. **Fat** digestion and absorption occurs exclusively in the small intestine, where as digestion and absorption of **carbohydrate** and **protein** occurs in both small and large intestine. In small intestine dietary carbohydrates and proteins are enzymatically broken down by pancreatic and brush border enzymes. The resulting hexoses and peptides or amino acids are then absorbed by small intestinal mucosa by specific active transport mechanism. In contrast carbohydrates and proteins entering the large intestine are digested by microbial action and produce VFA and NH_3, both this are absorbed by passive diffusion mechanism as the large intestine of most of the species don't have active transport mechanism for hexoses and amino acids. Dog and new born pig are exception to this generalization. The microbes responsible for fermentation in ruminant is consisting mainly of bacteria, fungi and protozoa. The majority of microbes particularly protozoa are anaerobic and therefore the main fermentation pathway are hydrolysis and anaerobic oxidation. Bacteria responsible for fermentation are of two types as **primary** and **secondary**. Primary bacteria are those that degrade the actual constituent of the diet so called **cellulolytic** or **amylolytic** depending on their action on cellulose or on starch. The fermentation end products of all carbohydrates are mainly acetic acid, propionic acid and butyric acid with a significant increase in the propionic acid. The fermentation of proteins yield theses acids together with valeric acids, isobutyric acids and isovaleric acids. These additional VFAs contribute less than 5%. Most of these VFAs produced are absorbed across the wall of fore stomach. These absorption occurs in the fashion butyric acid › propionic acid › acetic acid. These absorption is by passive diffusion and facilited diffusion. The principal gases produced during fermentation are CO_2 (60%), CH4 (30-40%), nitrogen, hydrogen sulphide, hydrogen and oxygen of trace amount. They are eliminated entirely by eructation.

The anatomy of avian alimentary canal differs most notably from that of mammal in the mouth area, presence of crop in oesophagus and presence of muscular stomach (**gizzard** or **ventriculus**). There are no soft palate in poultry. There is no teeth in poultry but salivary glands and taste buds are present. Small intestine is much more longer in herbivore birds than carnivorous. Parasitic infestation increase tract weight and length in chickens. Antibiotics decreases intestinal weight. Glandular stomach or proventriculus of birds function primarily in secretion. The muscular stomach or gizzard is highly specialized for grinding. Gizzard contain two pairs of muscles called musculi intermedii and musculi laterals.

Short Questions and Answers

1. **What is pre gastric fermenting and post gastric fermenting animals?**

Ans. **Pre gastric** fermenting animals are sheep, goat and cattle where fermentation takes place at proximal to gastric digestion. **Post gastric** fermenting animal is horse where fermentation takes place at distal part of digestive tract.

2. **What is prehension and what are prehensile organs in different animals?**

Ans. Prehension is the process of conveying of food to the mouth. Methods of prehension varies in animals but lip, teeth and tongue are the principal organs of prehension. **Dog and cat** use fore limb to hold food but pass in to mouth by head and jaw. **Horse** use mobile lips and incisor teeth for prehension, in **cattle and sheep** tongue is the principal prehensile organ but food get in by incisor teeth and dental pad. Lower lip is the prehensile organ of **pig.**

3. **What is mastication?**

Ans. **Mastication** is the mechanical break down of food in mouth. In domesticated animals the incisors are used to procure food. The molar teeth are used for grinding food into small particles.

Main purpose of mastication is to breakdown of food to provide a greater surface area for digestive juice. Important function of chewing is to mix food materials thoroughly with saliva. Such mixing ensures adequate lubrication of food bolus for its uninterrupted passage into the esophagus.

4. What is deglutination?

Ans. **Deglutination** or **swallowing** is the passage of food from mouth through pharynx and esophagus to the stomach. Movement of mouth and tongue are important in swallowing.

5. What is pseudoruminant?

Ans. Ruminant animals in which part of the stomach is absent is called **pseudoruminant**. Cammel is a ruminant where omasum is absent so it is called **pseudoruminant**.

6. What is migrating myoelectric complexes (MMC)?

Ans. During digestion of food particles, the large particles from stomach goes to distal part of intestine by the motility pattern is called **migrating myoelectric complexes (MMC).** This MMC is divided into three phases as **Phase I**: This is a quiescent period during which slow waves are present but no action potential is generated. **Phase II**: There is presence of intermittent action potential. **Phase III:** There is intense burst of spike accompanying each slow waves that results in strong gastric contraction. In carnivores but not in herbivores the MMC is interrupted on feeding resembling Phase II of MMC. The hormone **motilin** is involved in the initiation of MMC.

7. Mechanism of control of gastrointestinal function?

Ans. The integration of motor, secretory and absorptive events in the gastrointestinal tract is brought out by complex action of neural and endocrine systems.

Neural mechanism includes autonomic nervous system (ANS) and enteric nervous system (ENS). **ANS** include both sensory and motor component of sympathetic and parasympathetic division. Vagal and sacral nerves are main nerves responsible for gastrointestinal function. **ENS** is located in the wall of gastrointestinal tract on myeneric and submucosal plexus. These contain three types of neurons as motor neurons, inter neurons and sensory neurons.

Endocrine mechanism includes secretion of peptide hormones and amines that are released from the cells distributed throughout gastric, intestinal and pancreatic tissue on appropriate simulation. They are gastrin, secretin and cholecystokinin (CCK), pancreatic polypeptide, gastric inhibitory polypeptide, motilin, enteroglucagon and peptide Y which stimulate gastric acid secretion, increase gastrointestinal motility, stimulate pancreatic enzyme secretion, helps in growth of pancreatic tissue and gastrointestinal mucosa, where as secretin, gastric inhibitory polypeptide and enteroglucagon are three structurally homologous group which inhibit gastric acid secretion, **Ghrelin** is a hormone secreted from gastric fundus and is a growth hormone secretagogue. Apart from the potent GH releasing activity ghrelin actively participate in controlling energy balance, regulation of food intake, stimulation of appetite, gut motility, influence on reproduction, modulation of cardiovascular performances and immunological responses.

8. What is defecation?

Ans. It is the reflex act in which the feces are discharged from terminal colon and rectum. Distension of terminal colon and rectum is the normal stimulus for the reflex. Frightened animals frequently defecate. The efferent pathway of defecation reflex is cholinergic.

9. What are the functions of saliva?

Ans. A functional salivary unit is called salivon. Saliva performs many functions as, it facilitate mastication and deglutination which most important in herbivores, helps in regulation of body heat, for microbial digestion there should be a fluid medium and this fluid is solely from salivary gland as fore stomach has no secretory glands and the large quantities of acids produced by microbial digestion must be neutralized to preserve normal ruminal pH. Since saliva is rich in HCO_3- and PO_4^+ buffers, it neutralize the ruminal acids.

10. What is alkaline tide?

Ans. Mechanism by which hydrochloric acid is secreted from parietal cells to gastric lumen. Hydration of carbon dioxide in the parietal cells is responsible for the continuous production of H^+ and HCo_3^- ions. This reaction is catalyzed by carbonic anhydrase present in parietal cells. The H^+ ion produced in the parietal cells are transported to the gastric lumen by hydrogen pump by exchange of $1cl^-/1H^+$ as 1:1 fashion. The cl^- ions available to exchange with H^+ ion to gastric lumen is from blood in exchange with one HCo_3^- ion. So the metabolic alkalosis that occur during active acid secretion following a meal is called **alkaline tide**.

11. What is gastric mucosal barrier or gastric mucosal defence.

Ans. Because of H^+ ion concentration in the gastric lumen many times greater than that in the cell here must be diffusion of the ions to the surrounding tissue. But there are some mechanism of defence which is preventing this movement they are :

i) Electrical resistance of the cell membrane and surrounding area is high which resist the movement of H^+ ions.

ii) Mucus secreted by the neck chief cells which form a layer over mucosa.

iii) Bicarbonate ions secreted by the surface epithelium are trapped in the mucus gel so the H+ ions diffusing from lumen towards epithelium becomes neutralize and their concentration becomes zero.

iv) Endogenous prostaglandin acts as important gastric mucosal defence. Exact action how prostaglandin acts to save mucosa is not known but it is thought perhaps it increases HCO_3- secretion or mucosal blood flow.

12. What is restitution?

Ans. It is the process by which the superficial epithelium is restored within a minute after complete denudation by various injurious agents. This process involves active migrating mechanism of epithelium or viable cells to damaged area and spread over the denuded area and provide an effective barrier for mucosal injury. Some scientists called it as first line of defence against mucosal injury.

13. What is critical micellar concentration?

Ans. Normally for formation of micelle there must be present of minimum concentration of bile acid of 2mM in the jejunum. This concentration of bile acids are called **critical micellar concentration**.

14. What is the composition of feces?

Ans. Feces normally about $3/4^{th}$ of water and $1/4^{th}$ of solid and composed of 30% dead bacteria, 10-20% fat, 10-20% organic matter, 2-3% protein and 30% undigested roughage. Brown colour of feces is by stercobilin and urobilin. The odor of feces is caused by product of bacterial action which vary from person to person depending on their colonic bacteria and on the types of food eaten. The odoriferous product include indole, mercaptons, skatole and hydrogen sulphide.

15. What are the microbes responsible for fermentation?

Ans. The microbes responsible for fermentation is consisting mainly of bacteria, fungi and protozoa. The majority of microbes particularly protozoa are anaerobic and therefore the main fermentation pathway are hydrolysis and anaerobic oxidation. Bacteria responsible for fermentation are of two types as **primary** and **secondary**. Primary bacteria are those that degrade the actual constituent of the diet so called **cellulolytic** or **amylolytic** depending on their action on cellulose or on starch. Secondary bacteria are those which use their substrate to the end products of primary bacteria degradation and these group of bacteria include lactate utilizing propionate bacteria which produce propionate and methanogenic bacteria which produce methane. Action of ruminal fungi on fermentation is not known. The ruminal bacterias are normally **cellulolytic** and **amyloltyic**. Cellulolytic bacterias include Ruminococcus albus, butyrivibrio fibrisolvens, clostridium iochhi. Amyloltic bacterias include streptococcus bovis, rumonobacter amylophilus, prevotella ruminocola, succinimonas amylolytica, selenomonas ruminatium etc.

16. What is fermentation pathway?

Ans. This pathway involve 4 stages as

i) **First stage:** This stage involves hydrolysis of plant polysaccharides to their constituent monosaccharides and then there is conversion of these to fructose 1,6 biphosphate.

ii) **Second stage:** It involves EMP pathway for the anaerobic oxidation of fructose 1,6 biphosphate to pyruvate via phosphoenolpyruvate.

iii) **Third stage:** This stage involves the reaction that produce the final metabolites of fermentation. Phosenol pyruvate is the origin of the pathway leading to produce acetate, butyrate and propionate. Formate produce Methane and carbon dioxide.

iv) **Fourth stage:** It is the stage of microbial activity where there is synthesis of microbial compounds, particularly amino acid formation using above stages I to III intermediates. This stage involves the synthesis of microbial compounds such as protein, methane and also formation of butyrate and propionate by using the intermediates of stage I to III.

17. What is the fate of end products of fermentation?

Ans. The fermentation end products of all carbohydrates are mainly acetic acid, propionic acid and butyric acid with a significant increase in the propionic acid. The fermentation of proteins yield theses acids together with valeric acids, isobutyric acids and isovaleric acids. These additional VFAs contribute less than 5%. Most of these VFAs produced are absorbed across the wall of fore stomach. These absorption occurs in the fashion butyric acid › propionic acid › acetic acid. These absorption is by passive diffusion and facilited diffusion. During absorption of VFAs the butyric acid is metabolized to ketone body. These ketone bodies is used to synthesize C4-C14 chains of fatty acids in milk. About 30% of propionic acid is metabolized by the fore stomach wall to form lactic acid. In liver this lactate and remaining propionate is converted to glucose through kreb cycle. Propionate is the only VFA which is being used for glluconeogenesis. Acetate produced is taken upon by most of the body tissue to form Acetyl CoA and used in citric acid cycle. In mammary gland this acetate is used in synthesis of short and medium length fatty acid. Lactic acid produced by certain amylolytic bacterias during degradation of starch. These lactic acids is present in low concentration and is used by secondary bacterias to produce propionate. The principal gases produced during fermentation are CO_2 (60%), CH4 (30-40%), nitrogen, hydrogen sulphide, hydrogen and oxygen of trace amount. They are eliminated entirely by eructation.

18. How carbohydrate is digested in non ruminant?

Ans. Digestion of carbohydrate in monogastric animals starts from mouth. Monogastric diet normally consists of disaccharides as sucrose, lactose and polysaccharides like starches in grains. In mouth when food is chewed it mixed with saliva contain an enzyme ptyalin (á-amylase) secreted mainly by parotid gland. Amylase hydrolyse starch into disaccharides maltose and other small polymers of glucose that contain 3 to 9 glucose molecules. When food goes to stomach the activity of salivary amylase is blocked by the acid of gastric secretion. So next part of carbohydrate digestion occurs in small intestine. Digestion of carbohydrate in small intestine is called as **luminal phase**. Here hydrolysis of carbohydrate is by pancreatic amylases which is identical to amylase of saliva. Within 15-30 minutes after food goes from stomach to duodenum (duodanal lumen) they get mix with pancreatic amylase and hydrolyze the starch into trisaccharides and disaccharides but no free glucose is formed by pancreatic amylase hydrolysis. These tri and disaccharides are not absorbed directly by mucosa so they must further degraded into monosaccharides by the action of enzymes produced by intestinal mucosa or intestinal epithelial cells. This phase is called **mucosal phase**. The enzymes produced by intestinal epithelial cells are lactase, maltase, sucrose and á-dextrinase which are capable of splitting of disaccharides in to their respective monosaccharides. These enzymes are present in the lining of intestinal microvilli brush border. Finally these monosaccharides are absorbed by epithelial cells. Glucose and galactose are absorbed by an active transport system where as fructose is transported by diffusion system. Finally these monosaccharides which are water soluble are immediately absorbed to portal blood system for delivery to general body tissue.

19. How protein is digested in non ruminant?

Ans. Digestion of protein principally occurs in small intestine. But digestion of protein starts from stomach by action of pepsin. Pepsin the most important gastric enzyme which initiates the process of protein digestion usually providing only 10-20% of total protein digestion and convert the protein to proteoses, peptones and polypeptides. Most of the protein digestion occurs in the proximal part of small intestine i.e in duodenum and jejunum. The digestion of protein in this part is influenced by the enzymes from pancreatic secretion. These pancreatic proteases are of two types as i) **Endopeptidases** which include trypsinogen, chymotrypsinogen and elastase ii) **Exopeptidases** which include carboxypeptidase A & B. Exopeptidases breaks protein in to small peptides and amino acids. Further hydrolysis occurs at the intestinal brush boarder which secretes oligopeptidases and divide small peptides into corresponding amino acids and absorbed to the interior of intestinal cytoplasm or intestinal epithelial cells. Peptides of more than three amino acids can not be absorbed by the epithelium. These peptides and amino acids are absorbed to the cytoplasm by same mechanism like hexose transport by active transport system. Finally these absorbed peptides goes to portal blood system.

20. How Fat is digested in non ruminant?

Ans. First step of fat digestion is to break the fat globules into small size so that the water soluble digestive enzymes can act on the globule surface. Fat digestion in the intestinal lumen require both pancreatic and billiary secretion. Pancreatic lipase acts at the oil-water interface of the triglycerides and release fatty acid and β-monoglyceride. These products are water insoluble but are amphipaths i.e part of it is polar and water soluble and other part is non polar and water insoluble. The solubilization of the end products of lipase digestion is dependent on the action of bile acids. These acids acts as a detergent and bring the water insoluble material into solution by forming a negatively charge aggregate called micelle. The micelle is diffused to brush border epithelium. In the brush border epithelium the fatty acids and â-monoglyceride are esterified and associated with small amount of cholesterol, cholesterol esterase, certain apoproteins, phospholipid and finally form **chylomicron**. These chylomicrons are **water soluble micelle**. This water soluble micelle or chylomicron then diffuse to intestinal lymphatic system and finally to blood system, where as small quantities of short and medium chain fatty acids absorb directly to portal blood.

21. What are the movement of small intestine?

Ans. There are three types of intestinal motility are seen in small intestine. They are segmentation, pendular and peristalsis.

Segmentation: A mass of food lying in a length of intestine is divided into smaller pieces by constriction which occurs at regular intervals along the mass. The main result is to mix the food material with the digestive secretions and to repeatedly expose the mixture to the absorptive mucosa.

Pendular movement: This type of movement is the same as of segmentation and the differences in the expression are probably due to different experimental techniques.

Peristalsis: A progressive wave like movement that occurs involuntarily in hallow tubes of the body, specially the alimentary canal. It is characteristics of tubes possessing longitudinal and circular layers of smooth muscle fibers. Peristalsis is induced reflex by distension of the walls of the tube.

22. What are the movements of large intestine?

Ans. The movement of large intestine is very slow. At time the contractions may become powerful to bring about propulsion. **Colon** has three kinds of movements as reverse, peristalsis and sacculation. Peristalsis can occur any where in the colon. It is slow moving and serve to carry the ingesta down the colon in all herbivores, carnivores and omnivores. Reverse peristalsis is a common feature in many animals. **Cecum** is relatively small in carnivores and greatly developed in herbivores. In herbivores it function as fermentation place. Cecal movements are often very slow. Movements of cecum are essentially similar in all species and their function is to mix the ingesta.

23. What is regurgitation?

Ans. **Regurgitation** is the unique characteristic of the true ruminants like bovines, deers and giraffes and pseudoruminants like camels and llamas. It is most prominent in bovine and around 10 hours a day. This is seen when diet is of high roughages but the diet with low roughages or diet with finely grounded roughages reduces the rumination hour which is around 3 hours a day. The incidence of rumination has a circadian rhythm which is most commonly associated with the state of drowsiness. Highest incidence occurs during after noon and in the middle of the night. Many lactating ruminants ruminate while they are suckling their young or being milked. Rumination involves a stereotyped sequences of events called **regurgitation** which starts with inspiratory effort with the tongue and soft palate raised to block the buccal cavity and nasopharyngeal orifice respectively.

24. Bloat

Ans. When the eructation is inhibited, gas production by rumen microbes can not escape and create pressure which interfere the movement of diaphragm. So selection of proper food and antifoaming agents are used to control bloat. This bloat is mainly arises due to rumino reticular dysfunction. There are three factors that cause bloat. They are i) dietary factor ii) microbial factor and iii) animal factor.

25. Differences in alimentary tract of birds with mammals

Ans. The anatomy of avian alimentary canal differs most notably from that of mammal in the mouth area, presence of crop in oesophagus and presence of muscular stomach (gizzard or ventriculus). There are no soft palate in poultry. **There is no teeth in poultry but salivary glands and taste buds are present**. Small intestine is much more longer in herbivore birds than carnivorous. Parasitic infestation increase tract weight and length in chickens. Antibiotics decreases intestinal weight. Glandular stomach or proventriculus of birds function primarily in secretion. The muscular stomach or gizzard is highly specialized for grinding. Gizzard contain two pairs of muscles called musculi intermedii and musculi laterals. The small intestine of birds has a duodenum like that in mammals but beyond duodenum there is no sharp histological distinction into jejunum and ileum. The vestige of yolksac called **meckel's diverticulum** is found in the midway of small intestine. The cecum is paired and large intestine is shorter in birds. Liver in bird is bilobed. Gall bladder is present in chicken, duck and geese but not present in pigeon. The pancreas in bird is of three lobes.

Choose the Best Answer

1. End product of carbohydrate digestion in polygastric animal is

a) Glucose b) Amino acid
c) Fatty acid d) VFA

2. Progastric fermenting animal is

a) Sheep b) Dog
c) Cattle d) Horse

3. Intrinsic factor is secreted by

a) Chief cell b) Parietal cell
c) G cell d) Neck chief cell

4. Caecum and Colon are voluminous in

a) Horse b) Rabbit
c) Dog d) Pig

5. Large intestine of GI tract represent 75% of in which species

a) Sheep and Goat
b) Horse
c) Dog
d) Cattle

6. Stool shape is tablet like in sheep and goat because caecum is

a) Sacculated
b) Voluminous
c) Haustra like
d) Spheroid

7. Ratio of body length and intestine length in ox is

a) 1:8
b) 1:12
c) 1:20
d) 1:27

8. Prehensile organ in pig is

a) Teeth
b) Tounge
c) Lip
d) Jaw

9. Teeth helps for grinding is

a) Incisior
b) Canine
c) Molar
d) Pre-Molar

10. Vomiting does not occur in which species

a) Ruminant
b) Herbivorous
c) Carnivorous
d) Omnivorous

11. Saliva is isotonic in

a) Herbivorous
b) Carnivorous
c) Omnivorous
d) Ruminant

12. In non-ruminants microbial digestion takes place in

a) Stomach
b) Caecum & Colon
c) Rectum
d) Small intestine

13. Na+ ion is absorbed by

a) Active transport
b) Passive transport
c) Diffusion
d) Osmosis

14. Faces Contain how much part of water

a) ¼
b) ¾
c) ½
d) 1

15. Shape of omasum in ruminant is

a) Liver b) Kidney
c) Bean d) Zig zag

16. Secretory stomach in ruminant is

a) Rumen b) Reticulum
c) Omasum d) Abomesum

17. Primary bacteria in Ruminant is

a) Cellulolytic b) Amyllolytic
c) Methanogenic d) Lactate ferming

18. CH4 is produced by which type of bacteria

a) Primary b) Secondary
c) Both d) None

19. Gas produced by fermentation pathway is

a) CH4 b) CO_2
c) PEP d) a & b

20. CH4 and CO_2 produced in which phase of fermentation

a) 1st b) 2nd
c) 3rd d) 4th

21. Percentage of VFA (Acetate/ Propionate/ Butyrate) after fermentation of starch is

a) 55:25:15 b) 70:15:10
c) 45:45:10 d) 35:35:20

22. In pseudoruminant which part of the stomach is absent

a) Rumen b) Reticulum
c) Omasum d) Abomesum

23. Rumination occurs 10h/day in

a) Swine b) Bovine
c) Canine d) Feline

24. Percentage of CH_4 produced after fermentation is

a) 20-25% b) 30-40%
c) 50-60% d) 60%-70%

25. Bloat develops when animal fed with

a) Hay b) Silage
c) Grain d) Fresh legume

26. pH of Avian intestine is

a) 5.6-7.2 b) 2.3-5.0
c) 7-8 d) 4-7

27. Bile salt is absorbed in bird at

a) Caecum b) Rectum
c) Lower ileum d) Upper ileum

28. Bile salt is required for

a) Emulsification of fat b) Absorption of fat
c) Esterification of fat d) All

29. Which one of the following is ketone body

a) Acetone b) Acetic acid
c) β hydroxyl Butyrate d) All

30. Percentage of CO_2 produced after fermentation is

a) 20-25% b) 30-40%
c) 40-50% d) 60%-70%

31. VFA (Acetate/Propionate/Butyrate) produced after cellulose fermentation is

a) 70:15:10 b) 15:10:70
c) 10:70:15 d) 40:30:30

32. Which part of the polygastric stomach shows honey comb appearance

a) Rumen b) Reticulum
c) Omasum d) Abomesum

33. Papillae increases the

a) Tension b) Area
c) Permeability d) Motility

34. Which part of the polygastric stomach shows hexagonal ridge

a) Rumen b) Reticulum
c) Omasum d) Abomesum

35. Stomatostatin inhibit secretion of

a) Gastric b) Pancreatic
c) Hepatic d) All

36. Gastric motility is controlled by which nerve

a) Vagus b) Trochlear
c) Abducence d) Facial

37. Prehensile organ in pig is

a) Lower lip b) Upper lip
c) Teeth d) Tounge

38. Gall bladder is absent in

a) Horse b) Dog
c) Cat d) Cattle

39. If gall bladder is absent then bile stores in

a) Duodenum b) Liver
c) Pancrease d) All

40. Restitution means restoration of

a) Superficial epithelium b) Connective tissue
c) Muscular tissue d) Cardiac tissue

41. PH of pancrease in monogastric animal is

a) 6 b) 7
c) <8 d) >8

42. Process by which enzyme is secreted is called

a) Exocytosis b) Endocytosis
c) Pinocytosis d) Phagocytosis

43. Phase of the control of gastric function occurs when animal sees and smells food

a) Cephalic b) Gastric
c) Intestinal d) Interdigestive

44. Which type of meals would stay in the stomach for longest period of time

a) Meal high in lipids
b) Meal high in carbohydrates
c) Meal high in proteins
d) All would stay in the stomach about the same amount of time

45. Secretin is responsible for stimulating the secretion of _____ from the _____

a) Bile, gall bladder
b) Bicarbonate, pancreatic duct cells
c) Enzymes, pancreatic acinar cells
d) Water, pancreatic acinar cells

46. Which of the following is a function of the large intestine

a) Storage of undigested material until defecation
b) Absorption of water
c) Absorption of electrolytes
d) All of the above

47. Breakdown of proteins begins with secretions of

a) Salivary glands
b) Stomach
c) Pancreas
d) Small intestine

48. Breakdown of carbohydrates begins with secretions of the

a) Salivary glands
b) Stomach
c) Pancreas
d) Small intestine

49. Blood entering liver

a) Remains separate at all times (as far as arterial and venous blood is concerned)
b) Mixes with bile
c) Travels through a hepatic capillary network
d) Empties into spaces called sinusoids

50. Which of the following is not a part of the intestinal epithelial cell secretion

a) Trypsin
b) Maltase
c) Aminopeptidase
d) Lactase

51. Triglycerides travel through lymphatic vessels in the form of small particles called

a) Chylomicrons b) Lipid globules
c) Micelles d) Glycogen

52. Which hormone is released in the duodenum in response to acidic chime

a) Cholecystokinin b) Gastrin
c) Secretin d) Peptide

53. In the GI tract, layer responsible for absorption and secretions is

a) Mucosa b) Sub mucosa
c) Muscularis d) Serosa

54. Digestive enzyme produced in the salivary glands and pancreas is

a) Maltase b) Amylase
c) Pepsin d) Nuclease

55. Which keeps chyme in stomach until it reaches the right consistency to pass into small intestine

a) Esophageal sphincter b) Intrinsic sphincter
c) Cardiac sphincter d) Pyloric sphincter

56. Site where most of the chemical and mechanical digestion is carried out

a) Liver b) Stomach
c) Large intestine d) Small intestine

57. Parietal cells secrete

a) Serotonin b) Mucus
c) Pepsinogen d) Hydrochloric Acid

58. Cells at the base of fundic or oxyntic gland is

a) Chief cells b) Parietal cells
c) Argentaffin cells d) Goblet cells

59. Movement and flow of chemicals into the stomach is controlled by

a) Nervous system
b) Pancreas
c) Various digestive hormones
d) Both the nervous system and various digestive system hormones

60. Function of Ileum is to

a) Absorb nutrients
b) Absorb vitamin B_{12} and bile salts
c) To introduce bile and pancreatic juices
d) Absorb alcohol and aspirin

61. Liver does

a) Glycogen storage
b) Plasma protein synthesis
c) Bile production
d) Drug detoxification
e) All of the above

62. G.I tract is composed of how many layers

a) Two
b) Three
c) Four
d) Five

63. For formation of micelle the minimum concentration of bile acid in jejunum should be

a) 2mM
b) 4mM
c) 6mM
d) 8mM

64. Guttural pouch is present in

a) Horse
b) Cattle
c) Sheep
d) Goat

65. Which of the following is not comprise of the fore stomach

a) Reticulum
b) Rumen
c) Abomesum
d) Omasum

66. Vermiform appendix is a part of

a) Intestine
b) Stomach
c) Liver
d) Rectum

67. Ileum is a part of

a) Pelvic girdle
b) Pancrease
c) Large intestine
d) Small intestine

68. Pre-gastric fermentation are present in

a) Horse
b) Sheep
c) Cattle
d) Dog

69. Fat digestion and absorption exclusively occurs in

a) Small intestine
b) Large intestine
c) Both a & b
d) Stomach

70. Enzyme secreted from stomach is

a) Pepsin
b) Amylase
c) Maltase
d) All

71. Digestion of protein in non ruminants is started from

a) Mouth
b) Stomach
c) Small intestine
d) Large intestine

72. Salivary gland that secrete maximum saliva is

a) Parotid
b) Sub maxillary
c) Sub lingual
d) All secrete equal amount

73. In ruminant stomach food first goes to

a) Rumen
b) Reticulum
c) Omasum
d) Abomesum

74. Process by which animal catch food and carry to mouth is called

a) Prehension
b) Mastication
c) Deglutination
d) None

75. Fat digestion is facilitated by

a) Bile juice
b) Pancreatic juice
c) Liver juice
d) Gastric juice

76. Digestive juice that lacks enzyme but aid in digestion is

a) Chyle
b) Chyme
c) Bile
d) All

77. Organ which does not produce any digestive enzymes

a) Intestine b) Stomach
c) Liver d) Pacrease

78. Enzyme that is not secreted from pancrease is

a) Pepsin b) Trypsin
c) Peptidase d) Ribonuclease

79. Amount of saliva produce per day in human is

a) 200L b) 50L
c) 10L d) 2L

80. Which milk protein is acted upon by gastric enzyme

a) Casein b) Renin
ç) Pepsin d) Casinogen

81. HCl from stomach is secreted by

a) Zymogen cell b) Oxyntic cell
c) Kuffer cell d) Mucous cell

82. Honey comb like appearance is seen in which part of ruminant stomach

a) Rumen b) Reticulum
c) Omasum d) Abomesum

83. Brunner gland are found in

a) Stomach b) Duodenum
c) Ileum d) Pancrease

84 Action of pepsin requires a medium of

a) Alkaline b) Neutral
c) Acidic d) None

85. Endopeptidases are enzyme that acts on the substrate at the ________ of the molecule

a) Centre b) Inside
c) End d) Corner

86. Enzymes that acts at the ends of polypeptide chain is called

a) Endopeptidase b) Exopeptidase
c) Pepsinogen d) Zymogen

87. Animal has how many pairs of salivary gland

a) 3
b) 4
c) 5
d) 6

88. Salivary gland present below the ear is

a) Sub-maxillary
b) Sub-mandibular
c) Sub-lingual
d) Parotid

89. Enzyme present in saliva is

a) Ptyalin
b) Pepsin
c) Trypsin
d) Erepsin

90. Salivary enzyme requires which medium for its action

a) Acidic
b) Alkaline
c) Neutral
d) Salty

91. Method of food propulsion in oesophagus is called

a) Peristalsis
b) Antiperistlsis
c) Swallowing
d) Engulfing

92. Which of the following is of high in protein

a) Fruit
b) Water
c) Meat
d) Vegetables

93. Carbohydrates are used for

a) Energy
b) Repairing cells
c) Making muscles
d) Making skin

94. What is the solution used to detect sugar

a) Benedict's solution
b) Ethanol
c) Universal indicator
d) Biuret's solution

95. What is the solution used to test for proteins

a) Benedict's solution
b) Ethanol
c) Universal indicator
d) Biuret's solution

96. Proteins are needed by the body for

a) Energy
b) Growth and repair
c) Insulation
d) None of these

97. Nutrients present in the least amount in most of the foods is

a) Protein
b) Vitamins and minerals
c) Carbohydrates
d) Vat

98. Which of the following would be best for an athlete to eat before a race

a) Cheese sandwich
b) High protein bar
c) High carbohydrate bar
d) Hamburger

99. Which food is absorbed fastest

a) Protein
b) Sugar
c) Fat
d) Starch

100. Large food molecules are broken down to smaller molecules by

a) Water
b) Intestines
c) Stomach acid
d) Enzymes

101. Which of the following describe digestion

a) Breaking down large molecules into small molecules
b) Eating food
c) Absorbing food
d) Making large molecules from small molecules

102. Where does digested food go first

a) Heart
b) Brain
c) Bloodstream
d) Muscles

103. Which acid is produced in the stomach

a) Hydrochloric acid
b) Sulfuric acid
c) Citric acid
d) Digestion acid

104. Temperature where most of the enzymes work best is

a) 0°C
b) 37°C
c) 70°C
d) 100°C

105. What is the pH of the acid made in monogastric stomach

a) 1-2
b) 5-6
c) 8-9
d) 10-11

106. Glucose is most likely to be used in

a) Muscles b) Skin
c) Hair d) Nails

107. Which food in monogastric animal passes through the gut without being digested

a) Starch b) Fat
c) Protein d) Fibre

108. Undigested food that passes out of the body through the rectum is called

a) Vegetables b) Protein
c) Enzymes d) Faeces

109. Which of the following digestive organ part is absent in poultry

a) Teeth b) Soft palate
c) Both a & b d) None

110. Gall bladder is absent in which bird

a) Chicken b) Duck
c) Geese d) Pigeon

Answers

1. d	2. d	3. b	4. a	5.a	6. a	7. c	8. a	9. c	10. a
11. d	12. b	13. a	14. b	15. b	16. d	17. a&b	18. b	19. d	20. c
21. a	22. c	23. b	24. b	25. d	26. a	27. c	28. a	29. d	30. d
31 .a	32. b	33. b	34. b	35. a	36. a	37. a	38. a	39. a	40. a
41. d	42. a	43. a	44. a	45 .b	46. d	47. b	48. a	49. d	50. a
51. a	52. c	53. a	54. b	55. d	56. d	57. d	58. a	59. d	60. b
61. e	62. c	63. a	64. a	65. c	66. a	67. d	68. b	69. a	70. a
71. b	72. a	73. b	74. a	75. a	76. c	77. c	78. a	79. d	80. a
81. b	82. b	83. b	84. c	85. b	86. b	87. a	88. d	89. a	90. b
91. a	92. c	93. a	94. a	95. d	96. b	97. b	98. c	99. b	100. d
101. a	102. c	103. a	104. b	105. a	106. a	107. d	108. d	109. c	110. d

❑❑❑

CHAPTER-4

Endocrinology

Hormones are the chemical compound that is synthesized and secreted by a specialized group of cells or glands circulated by blood and exert its regulatory effect on target cells. The word hormone is derived from Greek word **"horman"** means arouse. The name of hormone was coined by **W. Baylis and E. Starling in 1902**. There are generally three classes of hormones as i) **Protein and polypeptides:** This class includes the hormones of anterior and posterior pituitary gland, pancreas and parathyroid gland ii) **Steroid:** This class includes the hormones of adrenal cortex (cortisol/androsterone), ovary (estrogen and progesterone), testes (testosterone) and placenta (estrogen and progesterone) and iii) **Derivative of amino acid tyrosine or amine hormones:** These hormones are secreted by thyroid (T3 and T4) and adrenal medulla (epinephrine and nor epinephrine). No hormones are there which are polysaccharides or nucleic acid. Water soluble hormones like peptides are dissolved in plasma and transport from their site of synthesis to target tissue where they diffuse out of the capillaries in to the interstitial fluid and goes to target cell. Where as steroid and thyroid hormones circulate in the blood mainly bound to the plasma proteins. So these protein bound hormones can not diffuse across the capillaries easily to target tissue and therefore biologically inactive until they dissociate from plasma protein. Protein and peptide (water soluble) hormones don't require carrier proteins for transport where as water insoluble hormones like steroid hormones require specific carrier protein. First step of hormone action is binding of hormone to specific receptor at the target cell. Receptors of different hormones present on different part of the cell. All hormone receptors are protein and have two functional domain as recognition domain and coupling domain. Recognition domain binds to hormone where as coupling domain regulate post binding biochemical events. The number of receptors on the target cell usually does not remain constant from day to day or even from minute to minute. After binding to receptor and forming hormone-receptor complex there is activation of receptor which initiates the hormone effect. The protein, polypeptide and amine hormones are water soluble which binds with the receptors on plasma membrane of the target cell and then exert their action by activation of intracellular enzymes (protein hormones) or by alteration of membrane permeability (neurotransmitters). The water insoluble steroid hormones and iodinated hormones (thyroid hormones) interact with nuclear, mitochondrial and cytoplasmic receptor and affect protein synthesis (steroid hormone) and gene transcription in the nucleus (thyroid hormone).

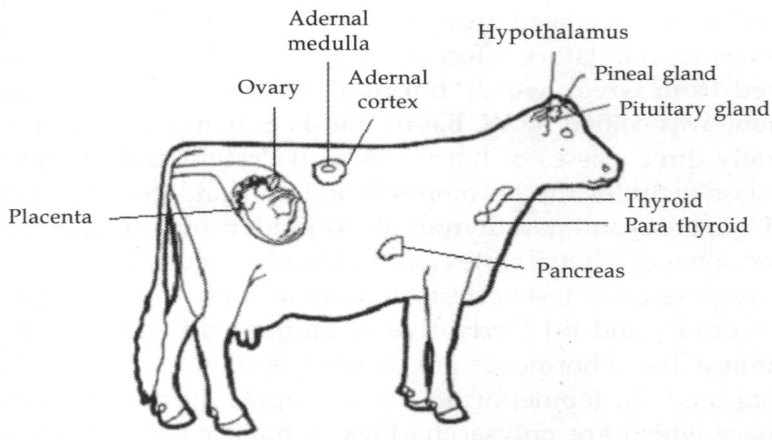

Endocrine glands of cattle

Pituitary gland was previously considered as master gland of body but now hypothalamus is called as **master gland** of body. The pituitary gland is also called as hypophysis. Physiologically pituitary gland is divided into two distinct parts as anterior pituitary called **adenohypophysis** and posterior pituitary called **neurohypophysis**. Between these two parts a small avascular sone is there called **pars intermedia** which is almost absent in human being but much larger and functional in some of the lower animals. Anterior pituitary has three parts as **pars distalis, pars tuberalis** and **pars intermedia**. Pars distalis is the largest part of adenohypophysis and contain five types of cells as **thyrotropes, gonadotropes, lactotropes, corticotropes** and **somatotropes**. These glandular cells secrete their respective hormones as thyrotropes (basophilic cells) secrete thyroid stimulating hormone, gonadotropes (basophilic cells) secrete gonadotropins (LH/FSH), lactotropes (eosinophillic cells) secrete prolactin, corticotropes secrete adreno corticotropic hormone (ACTH) and somatotropes (acdophillic cells) secrete somatotropins which is also called as growth hormone. The pars intermedia forms the junction between pars distalis and pars nervosa. Pars intermedia secrete **melanocyte stimulating hormone** (MSH) which regulate skin pigment in amphibians. Almost all the secretion by pituitary is controlled by either hormonal or neural signals from the hypothalamus. Secretion of anterior pituitary is controlled by hormones called hypothalamic releasing or hypothalamic inhibitory hormones or factors secreted within hypothalamus and then conducted anterior pituitary.

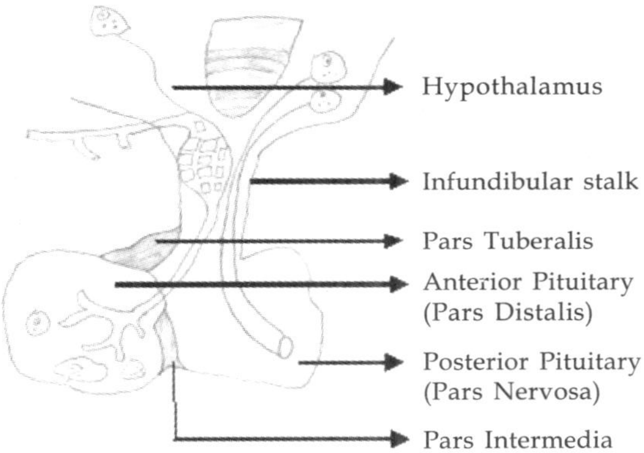

Hypothalamus - Pituitary Axis

All or most of the hypothalamic hormones are secreted at the nerve endings in the median eminence before being transported to the anterior pituitary. Electrical stimulation of this region excites these nerve ending and cause release of all hypothalamic hormones. Posterior pituitary is composed of mainly glial like cells called pituicytes. These pituicytes does not secrete hormone, they simply act as a supporting structure for large nerve fibers that originate in the supraoptic and paraventricular nuclei of hypothalamus and extend to pars nervosa of posterior pituitary. These axonic nerve fibers contain secretory granules of posterior pituitary hormones such as **ADH/vasopressin** and **oxytocin**. Both supraoptic and paraventricular nuclei synthesized both ADH and oxytocin. But ADH is formed primarily in the supraoptic nuclei where as oxytocin is formed primarily in paraventricular nuclei. Growth hormone exerts its effect on all most all the tissues of the body.

GH is otherwise called as **somatotropin** which is a single polypeptide chain with 191 amino acids and molecular weight of this hormone is 22kDa. Growth hormone has several metabolic effects including increasing rate of protein synthesis in most cells of the body, increase mobilization of fatty acids from adipose tissue and decrease utilization of glucose throughout the body and increase in deposition of glycogen in the cell. Gonadotrpins include **follicle stimulating hormone (FSH) and luteinizing hormone (LH)**. Some times prolactin is also included among gonadotropins because in certain species it stimulate corpus luteum functioning. Both FSH and LH have carbohydrate moieties attached so both termed as glycoproteins but prolactin in contrast is a polypeptide hormone. FSH regulates the development, growth, pubertal maturation and reproductive processes of the body. FSH and luteinizing hormone (LH) act synergistically in reproduction. Prolactin regulates lactation. Prolactin stimulates mammary gland to produce milk. It cause enlargement of mammary gland and increases the production of milk. It stimulate proliferation of oligodendrocyte precursor cells. **Thyroid gland** is the first endocrine gland to appear in the developing individual. It is one of the largest gland of body and secrete two major hormones as thyroxine (T_4) and triiodothyronine (T_3) and calcitonin. Thyroxine is composed of 93% of thyroid secretion and just 7% is triiodothyronine. Metabolically T_3 is more active than T_4. Function of both the hormones are qualitatively same but they differ in rapidity and intensity of action. T3 is four times more potent than T_4 but T_3 is present in the blood much smaller quantity. Thyroid hormone increases basal metabolic rate (BMR) 60-100% above than normal in excess secretion and 40% below normal in less secretion. There are normally four parathyroid glands which are located behind to thyroid glands at the upper and lower poles.

Short Questions and Answers

1. **What hormone and its classification?**

Ans. **Hormones** are the chemical compound that is synthesized and secreted by a specialized group of cells or glands circulated by blood and exert its regulatory effect on target cells. The word hormone is derived from Greek word **"horman"** means arouse. The name of hormone was coined by **W. Baylis and E. Starling in 1902**. There are generally three classes of hormones as :

i) **Protein and polypeptides:** This class includes the hormones of anterior and posterior pituitary gland, pancreas and parathyroid gland.

ii) **Steroid:** This class includes the hormones of adrenal cortex (cortisol/androsterone), ovary (estrogen and progesterone), testes (testosterone) and placenta (estrogen and progesterone)

iii) **Derivative of amino acid tyrosine or amine hormones:** These hormones are secreted by thyroid (T3 and T4) and adrenal medulla (epinephrine and nor epinephrine).No hormones are there which are polysaccharides or nucleic acid.

2. How hormones are transported in blood?

Ans. Water soluble hormones like peptides are dissolved in plasma and transport from their site of synthesis to target tissue where they diffuse out of the capillaries in to the interstitial fluid and goes to target cell. Where as steroid and thyroid hormones circulate in the blood mainly bound to the plasma proteins. So these protein bound hormones can not diffuse across the capillaries easily to target tissue and therefore biologically inactive until they dissociate from plasma protein. Protein and peptide (water soluble) hormones don't require carrier proteins for transport where as water insoluble hormones like steroid hormones require specific carrier protein.

3. What is the mechanism of action of peptide hormones?

Ans. **Action of peptide hormones is through second messenger mechanism.** The most common second messenger system involves is cyclic AMP (cAMP). The binding of water soluble hormones to their plasma membrane receptor results in generation of one or more second messenger. These second messenger then regulate the intracellular events that constitute the target cell response. After binding of hormone to receptor on the surface of plasma membrane, the hormone-receptor complex stimulate G-protein which is coupled to receptor. Stimulated G-protein activate adenyl cyclase a membrane bound enzyme that catalyze the conversion of small amount of cytoplasmic ATP to cAMP inside cell. cAMP then activate protein kinase which phosphorylates specific protein in the cell triggering biochemical reactions (gene activation, secretion, ion transport, cell growth, cell respiration, carbohydrate and fat metabolism etc) that ultimately leads to cell's response to hormone. Example of hormones that act through adenyl cyclase–cAMP second messenger system are ACTH, FSH, LH, HCG, vasopressin (epithelial cell), calcitonin etc. The other second messenger system for peptide hormone action are :

i) **Phospholipid second messenger system**

Some hormones after binding to receptor activate the enzyme phospholipase C attached to the inside projection of the receptors. This enzyme catalyze the break down of phosphatidyl inoistol biphosphate (PIP2) on cell membrane into two second messenger as inositol triphosphate (IP3) and diacyl glycerol (DAG). The IP3 mobilize calcium ion from mitochondria and endoplasmic reticulum and calcium ion show its own second messengeric effect such as smooth muscle contraction. Where as DAG activate protein kinase C which phosphorylates number of proteins leading to cells response. Example of hormones that act through phospholipid second messenger system are oxytocin, vasopressin (vascular smooth muscle), thyroid releasing hormone, gonadotropin releasing hormone etc.

ii) **Calcium-calmodulin second messenger pathway**

This is second messenger system which operates in response to the entry of calcium ion into the cell. This calcium ion may be initiated by change in membrane potential that opens calcium channel or hormone interact with membrane receptor that open calcium channel.

4. What is the mechanism of action of steroid hormone and thyroid hormone?

Ans. The steroid hormones are specially secreted by ovaries, testes and adrenal cortex that cause synthesis of proteins in target cell. These proteins then function as enzymes, transport proteins or structural proteins which in turn provide other functions of cell. The sequence of events of steroid hormone action is i) the steroid hormone enters the cytoplasm of the cell where it binds with specific receptor protein, ii) the combined receptor protein and hormone diffuses in to he nucleus, iii) the combination binds at specific points on the DNA strand in the chromosome which activate the transcription process of specific genes to form m RNA, iv) mRNA formed in nucleus comes out to cytoplasm and reaches to ribosomes and activates them to produce large number of proteins which cause physiological responses in the target cell. Thyroid hormones act in the similar way as steroid hormone but their receptors are in the nucleus. Thyroid hormones increase transcription by specific genes in the nucleus. These hormones first bind to the receptor protein in the nucleus and cause gene transcription that shows physiological responses in target cell.

5. **What are different parts of pituitary gland?**

Ans. Pituitary gland is divided into two distinct parts as anterior pituitary called **anterior pituitary (adenohypophysis)** and posterior pituitary called **anterior pituitary (neuro-hypophysis)**. Between these two parts a small avascular sone is there called **pars intermedia** which is almost absent in human being but much larger and functional in some of the lower animals. Anterior pituitary has three parts as **pars distalis, pars tuberalis** and **pars intermedia.** Posterior pituitary consists of two parts i.e **infundibulum or pituitary stalk** and **pars nervosa or neural lobe.**

6. **What are the hormones secreted by pituitary gland?**

Ans. Pituitary gland is divided into two distinct parts as anterior pituitary called **anterior pituitary (adenohypophysis)** and posterior pituitary called **anterior pituitary (neuro-hypophysis)**. Anterior pituitary has three parts as **pars distalis, pars tuberalis** and **pars intermedia**. Pars distalis is the largest part of adenohypophysis and contain five types of cells as **thyrotropes, gonadotropes, lactotropes, corticotropes** and **somatotropes**. These glandular cells secrete their respective hormones as thyrotropes (basophilic cells) secrete thyroid stimulating hormone, gonadotropes (basophilic cells) secrete gonadotropins (LH/FSH), lactotropes (eosinophillic cells) secrete prolactin, corticotropes secrete adreno corticotropic hormone (ACTH) and somatotropes (acdophillic cells) secrete somatotropins which is also called as growth hormone. Pars tuberalis is an upward extension of adenohypophysis and attached to infundibulum. The pars intermedia forms the junction between pars distalis and pars nervosa. **Pars intermedia** secrete **melanocyte stimulating hormone** (MSH) which regulate skin pigment in amphibians. Posterior pituitary consists of two parts i.e **infundibulum or pituitary stalk and pars nervosa or neural lobe**. Posterior pituitary secrete two hormones as oxytocin and vasopressin (ADH). The bodies of the cells that secrete these hormones are not located in the pituitary gland but are large neurons called **magnocellular neurons** located in the **supraoptic and paraventricular nuclei** of hypothalamus. The hormones after synthesis in hypothalamus are transported to posterior pituitary and stored there. At the time of necessary the hormones are released from posterior pituitary.

7. How hypothalamus control pituitary secretion?

Ans. Almost all the secretion by pituitary is controlled by either hormonal or neural signals from the hypothalamus. Secretion of anterior pituitary is controlled by hormones called hypothalamic releasing or hypothalamic inhibitory hormones or factors secreted within hypothalamus and then conducted anterior pituitary. In **anterior pituitary** these factors acts on glandular cells to control their secretion. Where as the secretion of **posterior pituitary** is controlled by nerve signals that originate in hypothalamus and terminate in posterior pituitary. The major hypothalamic releasing and inhibitory hormones are thyrotropin releasing hormone (TRH) which causes release of thyroid stimulating hormone, corticotropin releasing hormone (CRH) which cause release of adrenocorticotropin which is also called as **corticotrophin,** growth hormone releasing hormone (GHRH) which cause release of growth hormone, growth hormone release inhibiting hormone (GIH) also called as **somatostatin** which inhibits the release of growth hormone, gonadotropin releasing hormone (GnRH) which cause the release of two gonadotropins as LH and FSH, prolactin releasing hormone (PRL) which stimulate to secrete prolactin and Prolactine release inhibiting hormone (PIH) that inhibit the secretion of prolactin. **Magnocellular neurons** located in the **supraoptic and paraventricular nuclei** of hypothalamus secrete two hormones as oxytocin and vasopressin (ADH). The hormones after synthesis in hypothalamus are transported to posterior pituitary and stored there. At the time of necessary the hormones are released from posterior pituitary.

8. What is growth homone and its function?

Ans. Growth hormone (GH) is otherwise called as **somatotropin** which is a single polypeptide chain with 191 amino acids and molecular weight of this hormone is 22kDa. All the anterior pituitary hormones beside growth hormone (GH) exert their principal effects by stimulating target glands. GH exerts its effect on all most all the tissues of the body. It causes growth of all tissues of body that are capable of growing, It promotes increase in size of the cells and increase mitosis. Growth hormone has several metabolic effects including increasing rate of protein synthesis in most cells of the body, increase mobilization of fatty acids from adipose tissue and decrease utilization of glucose throughout the body and increase in deposition of glycogen in the cell.

9. What is gigantism?

Ans. Gigantism is the condition due to hypersecretion of GH in childhood or in pre adult life before the fusion of epiphysis of bones with shaft. This hyper secretion of GH may because of tumor of acidophil cells in the anterior pituitary because of which these cells become excessively active so large quantities of GH are produced. In this condition there will be over growth of the affected individual, limbs are disproportionately long, affected individuals are hyperglycemic and they develop glycosuria and diabetes mellitus. Tumor of pituitary gland cause constant headache and visual disturbances. In most of cases of gigantism hypopituitarism develops which leads to burning out of cells of anterior pituitary or destruction of anterior pituitary.

10. What is acromegaly?

Ans. This condition develops due to hyper secretion of GH in adult after the fusion of epiphysis with shaft of the bone. This hypersecretion of GH is due to tumor of anterior pituitary involving acidophilic cells. In this condition there is enlargement, thickening and broadening of bones particularly in the extrimities of the body. Broadning of nose, thickening of lips, thickening and wrinkles on fore head, protrusion of lower jaw. The face with these features are called acromegalic or **guerrillea shape**. There is enlargement of hand and feets, over growth of body hairs, visceral organs like lungs, thymus, heart, liver and spleen are enlarged. Thyroid, parathyroid and adrenal glands show hyperactivity. There is hyperglycemia and glucosuria resulting diabetes mellitus and hypertension. In animal there is over growth of connective tissues, increase in growth of bones and enlargement of viscera.

11. What is function of ADH/ vasopressin?

Ans. Vasopressin increases water reabsorption from distal convoluted tubule and collecting ducts of the kidney. Both DCT and collecting ducts are totally impermeable to water in absence of ADH. ADH cause special structural changes in the membrane of the tubular epithelial cells which provides many temporary new pores that cause free diffusion of water through pores. Vasopressin causes constriction of the arteries in all parts of the body. Due to vasoconstriction the blood pressure is increased.

12. What is diabetes insipidus?

Ans. The deficiency of ADH causes **diabetes insipidus**. This disease is characterized by excessive secretion of water through urine. Symptoms of diabetes insipidus are polyurea, polydipsia, dehydration and hyperosmolarity.

13. How Thyroid hormone is synthesized?

Ans. Iodine and Tyrosine are essential for the formation of Thyroid hormone. Iodine and Tyrosine are consumed through diet. Iodine is converted to iodide and absorbed to GI tract. Tyrosine is also absorbed through GI tract. There are various steps for formation of thyroid hormones. They are

i) Thyroglobulin secretion

ii) Iodide trapping (Iodine pump)

iii) Oxidation of iodide

iv) Iodination of Tyrosine

i) **Thyroglobulin secretion:** Thyroid gland is composed of large numbers of closed follicles filled with secretory substances called **colloid**. The colloid of thyroid gland synthesize and secrete a large glycoprotein molecule in to the follicle called **thyroglobulin**, with a molecular weight of 335kDa. Each molecule of thyroglobulin contains about 75-100 tyrosine amino acids which combine with iodine to form thyroid hormone.

ii) **Iodide trapping:** Iodine is transported actively from the blood in to the folecullar cells of thyroid glandular cells. The basal membrane of the thyroid cells has the specific ability to pump iodine actively to the interior of the cell. This is called **iodide trapping**.

iii) **Oxidation of iodide ion:** Iodide has to be oxidized to iodine which is capable of combining with tyrosine to form thyroid hormone. The oxidation of iodide to iodine occurs inside cell and promoted by enzyme **thyroid peroxidase**.

iv) **Iodination of Tyrosine or Organification of thyroglobulin:** The combination of iodide with tyrosine is called **Iodination**. It takes place in the follicle within thyroglobulin. First iodine is released in follicular cavity and bind with thyroglobulin. Binding of iodine with tyrosine in thyroglobulin is called **organification of thyroglobulin**. Binding of iodine with tyrosine is acclerated by enzyme **iodinase.** Iodination of tyrosine occurs in several stages. Tyrosine is iodized first in to monoiodotyrosine (MIT) or diiodotyrosine (DIT). One DIT combine with one MIT to form triiodothyronine (T_3), where as two DIT combine to form tetraiodo thyronine (T_4)/thyroxine. Out of the hormones produced in thyroid gland thyroxine contributes about 90% and T_3 contribute about 9-10% of total thyroid hormone. Biological potency of T_3 is more than T_4.

14. What is function of thyroid hormone (TH)?

Ans. TH increases metabolic activity of cells of the body, increases Basal metabolic rate (BMR) 60-100% above than normal in excess secretion and 40% below normal in less secretion, activate protein metabolism by increasing translation and transcription, increases activity of intracellular enzymes, increase carbohydrate metabolism by increasing glucose uptake by cell, increasing absorption of glucose by GI tract and bynhance glycolysis and gluconeogenesis, decreases fat stores of the body, increases fat metabolism, increases free fatty acids concentration in plasma but decrease the concentration of cholesterol, phospholipids and triglycerides, increases formation of many enzymes: So there is shown of vitamin deficiency during excess secretion of thyroid as vitamins are utilized for formation of enzymes, increase in TH decreases body weight where as decrease in TH increase body weight. This increase in body weight don't occur always because TH increase appetite which counter balance metabolic rate, increase heat production in body due to increase in BMR so temperature of body increase, TH is important for growth and development of brain during fetal life and few years after postnatal life, increase production of RBC and blood volume, in heart TH increase heart rate, increase cardiac strength, increase cardiac output, increase cardiac blood volume, increase cardiac force of contraction, increase systolic pressure and decrease diastolic pressure so pulse pressure is constant and increase in BP, increase rate and force of respiration, hypothyroidism cause diarrhea and hyperthyroidism cause constipation as TH cause motility of GI tract, cause growth and development of brain, increase muscle to work with more vigor so excess secretion cause weakness of muscle due to catabolism of protein called **thyrotoxic myopathy**. Lack of TH cause muscle to become sluggish. Hypersecrtion of TH cause excessive stimulation of CNS so person feels tired and feel sleepy but cann't sleep as of stimulatory effect of TH on neuron, lack of TH decrease libido in male leads to impotence.

15. What is Grave's disease?

Ans. It is an auto immune disease where the thyroid stimulating auto antibodies (B-TSAB) produced by B- lymphocytes which activate TSH receptors and increase the secretion of thyroid hormone.

16. What are symptoms of hyperthyroidism?

Ans. Intolerance to heat because the body has already produces lots o heat due to increased basal metabolic rate, increased sweating due to vasodilation, weight loss due to fat mobilization, high state of excitability, nervousness, inhibits to sleep, extreme anxiety or worry. These symptoms are due to excessive stimulation of neurons of central nervous system, diarrhoea due to increase in gastro intestinal motility, enlargement of thyroid gland called toxic goiter. This is due to tumor in the gland and increase in number of hormone secreting cells,there is exopthalamus (protrusion of eye ball). This protrusion of eyeball stretches the optic nerve and cause damage to optic nerve resulting blindness. Due to protrusion the eye lids can not be closed completely while blinking or during sleep. Cause of protrusion of eye ball is edematous swelling of retro-orbital tissues and degenerative changes in extra ocular muscles.

17. What is myxedema?

Ans. Myxedema develops due to hypothyroidism in adults. Symptom of myxedema is edematous appearance throughout the body, swelling of face, bagginess under the eyes, **non pitting type edema**: It means when this edema is pressed it does not makes pit and the edema is hard. This is because of accumulation of proteins, **Artherosclerosis**: This is because of increased content of cholesterol in plasma. Because of this the cholesterol is deposited on the wall of the blood vessels causing artherosclerosis.

18. What is general symptoms of hypothyroidism?

Ans. Fatigue and muscular sluggishness, polymenorrhoea, menorrhagia, decreased cardiovascular function such as i) reduced heart rate ii) decrease in force of contraction of heart iii) decrease in cardiac output iv) decreased blood volume, Increased body weight, constipation, mental sluggishness, decreased hair growth, scaliness of skin, husky voice.

19. What is cretinism?

Ans. It is caused by extreme hypothyroidism during fetal life. Cause of cretinism may be due to congenital absence of thyroid gland, genetic disorder and lack of iodine in diet. **Symptoms** of cretinism are: A newborn baby with thyroid deficiency may appear normal at birth but few weeks after birth the baby starts signs like sluggish movement, cracking sound while crying, failure of body growth (stunted growth), mental retardation, tongue become so big that it hangs down with dripping of saliva. The big tongue obstructs swallowing and breathing including a characteristic guttural breathing.

20. What is goiter and types of goiter?

Ans. Goiter means enlargement of thyroid gland. This can occur both in hypothyroidism and hyperthyroidism. **Goiter in hyperthyroidism** is otherwise called as **toxic goiter**. Here the size of the gland increases because of increase in number of hormone secreting cells because of which the hormone level also increases to vary great extent. **Goiter in hypothyroidism** is otherwise called as **nontoxic goiter**. Here the size of the gland increases but secretion is reduced. This type of goiter is of two types i) Endemic goiter and ii) Idiopathic/non toxic goiter. **Endemic goiter/colloid goiter** is also called as **iodine deficiency goiter**. It is due to lack of iodine intake. Here there is lack of iodine which prevent production of both T3 and T4 but there is more TSH from anterior pituitary which stimulate thyroid cell to secrete more thyroglobulin in to the tonsil so gland grow larger. **Idiopathic/non toxic goiter** is enlargement of thyroid gland. Exact cause is not known. But it is suggested that patient is affected first by **thyroiditis** which reduce the synthesis of hormone but there is secretion of TSH to gland which cause increase in size of gland.

21. What is function of parathyroid hormone?

Ans. The primary function of parathromone is to maintain the blood calcium and phosphate level within the crucial range of 9-11mg%. Parathromone maintain blood calcium level by increasing the reabsorption of calcium from bone, by decreasing the excretion of calcium through or by kidney and increase renal phosphate excretion and by increasing absorption of calcium from gastro intestinal tract.

22. What is function of calcitonin

Ans. Primary stimulus for calcitonin secretion is increased plasma calcium ion. Calcitonin plays an important role in the maintenance of blood calcium level along the parathromone. It decreases blood calcium level and thereby counter acts the action of parathromone. Calcitonin reduces the blood calcium by action on bone, kidney and intestine. Calcitonin facilitate deposition of calcium on bones. Calcitonin increases the excretion of calcium through urine by inhibiting reabsorption of calcium from the tubules. Calcitonin prevents the absorption of calcium from intestine in to the blood.

23. What is function of follicle stimulating hormone (FSH)?

Ans. FSH regulates the development, growth, pubertal maturation, and reproductive processes of the human body. In both males and females, FSH stimulates the maturation of germ cells. In males, FSH induces sertoli cells to secrete inhibin and stimulates the formation of sertoli-sertoli tight junctions (zonula occludens). In females, FSH initiates follicular growth, specifically affecting granulosa cells. With the concomitant rise in inhibin B, FSH levels then decline in the late follicular phase.

24. What is function of luteinizing hormone (LH)?

Ans. **LH** is a hormone produced by the anterior pituitary gland. In the female, an acute rise of LH i.e the LH surge triggers ovulation and corpus luteum development. In the male, where LH had also been called **interstitial Cell stimulating hormone (ICSH)**, it stimulates leydig cell for production of testosterone.

25. What are gastro intestinal hormones?

Ans. There are number of gastrointestinal hormones. They are

Gastrin is secreted fro the G-cells of islets of langerhans of pancreas and also from duodenum.

Secretin is secreted from duodenum and jejunum part of small intestine.

Cholecystokinin is secreted from duodenum and also from jejunum.

Ghrelin is secreted mainly by the stomach and, to a less degree, by various organs: intestine, pancreas, kidney, hypothalamus, pituitary gland. Ghrelin secretion increases under fasting conditions and falls after food intake.

Pancreozymin is secreted from duodenum and jejunum part of the small intestine. It helps in pancreatic secretion, that is, pancreatic lipase, trypsin etc. enzymes are secreted under the control of that hormone.

Neurotensin is only secreted from ileum of small intestine and prohibits the motor activity of stomach.

Enterocrinin is secreted from intestinal mucosa and controls the secretion of intestinal hormones from intestinal mucosa.

Villikinin is secreted from small intestine and helps to move villi and thus helps in absorption of digested food materials.

Enteroglucagon is secreted from pancreas, ileum of small intestine and colon of large intestine. It helps in the growth of intestinal mucosa.

Motilin is secreted from enterochromaffin cells of gut. This hormone stimulates the secretion of pepsin and also helps in the movement of different part of Gastro-intestinal tract.

Duocrinin is secreted from the mucosal part of duodenum. It helps to secrete mucous from Bruner's glands (Bruner's glands are tubular branched glands located in the duodenum and secrete mucous along with bicarbonates, also protect small intestine from acidic chime).

Glucagon-like peptide-1 (GLP-1) is secreted by the digestive tract, mainly the ileum and the colon, secretion stimulated by food intake.

Enterostatin is an anorectic pentapeptide, formed in the lumen of the small intestine from the pancreatic procolipase under the influence of digestive enzymes.

26. What are pancreatic hormones?

Ans. Pancreas is an exocrine gland has several hundred thousand clusters of cells called islets of langerhans. The islets are endocrine tissue containing four types of cells. They are α

cells (22% of the pancreatic hormone-secreting cells) which secrete glucagon, β **cells** (70% of the pancreatic hormone-secreting cells) which secrete insulin and **amylin, d cells** that secrete somatostatin and g **cells** secrete a polypeptide of unknown function.

27. What are the functions of glucagon?

Ans. Glucagon helps maintain the level of glucose in the blood by binding to glucagon receptor on hepatocytes causing the liver to release glucose stored in the form of glycogen. Glucagon also regulates the rate of glucose production through lipolysis. Insulin and glucagon have reciprocal roles. Insulin promotes the storage of glucose, fatty acids and amino acids whereas glucagon stimulates mobilization of these constituents from storage into the blood. Glucagon secretion is stimulated by decreased blood glucose levels, infection, cortisol, exercise and large protein meals. Glucagon stimulates glycogen breakdown in the liver, inhibits glycogen synthesis and facilitates glucose release into the blood. Excess glucagon can result from tumors of the pancreatic á cells and a mild diabetes seems to result. Some cases of uncontrolled diabetes are also characterized by high glucagon levels suggesting that low blood insulin levels are not always the only cause in some diabetes cases.

28. What is the action of insulin on cells?

Ans. There are different actions of insulin on cells as increased glycogen synthesis, increased fatty acid synthesis, increased esterification of fatty acids, decreased proteolysis, decreased lipolysis, decreased gluconeogenesis, decreased autophagy, increased amino acid uptake, increased potassium uptake, Increase in the secretion of hydrochloric acid by Parietal cells in the stomach.

29. What is diabetes mellitus?

Ans. **Diabetes mellitus** is a condition in which the body either does not produce enough or does not properly respond to insulin, the hormone produced in the pancreas. Insulin enables cells to absorb glucose in order to turn it into energy. This causes glucose to accumulate in the blood, leading to various potential complications.

Many types of diabetes are recognized: The main three are:

Type 1: also called as **childhood onset diabetes**, juvenile diabetes and insulin dependent diabetes mellitus (IDDM). It results from the body's failure to produce insulin. Presently most persons with type 1 diabetes take insulin injections.

Type 2: also called as **adult onset diabetes**, obesity related diabetes and non insulin dependent diabetes mellitus (NIDDM). It results from insulin resistance, a condition in which cells fail to use insulin properly, sometimes combined with absolute insulin deficiency.

Gestational diabetes: Pregnant women who have never had diabetes before but who have high blood sugar (glucose) levels during pregnancy are said to have gestational diabetes.

30. What are symptoms of diabetes mellitus?

Ans. In diabetes mellitus, there is excessive sweet urine called as glycosuria. There is polyurea (frequent urination), polydipsia (increased thirst) and polyphagia (increased hunger). Symptoms may develop quite rapidly (weeks or months) in type 1 diabetes, particularly in children. However, in type 2 diabetes symptoms usually develop much more slowly and may be subtle or completely absent. Type 1 diabetes may also cause a rapid significant weight loss and irreducible mental fatigue. All of these symptoms except weight loss can also manifest in type 2 diabetes in patients whose diabetes is poorly controlled, although unexplained weight loss may be experienced at the onset of the disease.

31. What is function of pineal gland?

Ans. **Pineal gland** (also called the **pineal body, epiphysis cerebri, epiphysis** or **third eye**) is a small endocrine gland in the vertebrate brain. It produces **melatonin** a hormone that affects the modulation of wake/sleep patterns and photoperiodic (seasonal) functions. It is shaped like a tiny pine cone and is located near to the center of the brain, between the two hemispheres, tucked in a groove where the two rounded thalamic bodies join.

Function of melatonin

Melatonin is a derivative of the amino acid tryptophan, which also has other functions in the central nervous system. The production of melatonin by the pineal gland is stimulated by darkness and inhibited by light. Photosensitive cells in the retina detect light and directly signal the suprachiasmatic nucleus (SCN), entraining its rhythm to the 24-hour cycle in nature. Fibers project from the SCN to the paraventricular nuclei (PVN), which relay the circadian signals to the spinal cord and out via the sympathetic system to superior cervical ganglia (SCG) and from there into the pineal gland. The functions of melatonin in humans are not clear; it is commonly prescribed for the treatment of circadian rhythm sleep disorders. The compound **pinoline** is also produced in the pineal gland, it is one of the α-carbolines. In animals, the pineal gland appears to play a major role in sexual development, hibernation, metabolism and seasonal breeding. Modern birds and reptiles have been found to express the phototransducing pigment melanopsin in the pineal gland. Avian pineal glands are believed to act like the suprachiasmatic nucleus in mammals.

32. What is function of prostaglandins?

Ans. Prostaglandins are like hormones in that they act as chemical messengers. They are biochemically synthesized from the fatty acid, arachidonic acid.

Functions of Prostaglandins

There are a variety of physiological effects like

i) Activation of the inflammatory response, production of pain and fever. When tissues are damaged, white blood cells flood to the site to try to minimize tissue destruction. Prostaglandins are produced as a result.

ii) Blood clots form when a blood vessel is damaged. A type of prostaglandin called thromboxane stimulates constriction and clotting of platelets. Conversely, PGI2, is produced to have the opposite effect on the walls of blood vessels where clots should not be forming.

iii) Certain prostaglandins are involved with the induction of labor and other reproductive processes. PGE2 causes uterine contractions and has been used to induce labor.

iv) Prostaglandins also increase blood flow in kidneys and leukotriens promote constriction of bronchi associated with asthma.

33. What is function of thymus gland?

Ans. The **thymus gland** is a pink-grey organ that is known as **sweetbreads**. It has two lobes, each divided into lobules by a partitian called a septum or wall. Each lobule consists of a densely packed outer cortex center medulla. In the two thymic lobes, lymphocyte precursors from the bone-marrow become thymocytes and subsequently mature into T cells. Once mature, T cells emigrate from the thymus and constitute the peripheral T cell repertoire responsible for directing many facets of the adaptive immune system. Loss of the thymus at an early age through genetic mutation or surgical removal results in severe immunodeficiency.

34. What is panhypopituitarism?

Ans. This term indicates the decrease secretion of all the anterior pituitary hormones or even absent. This decrease in secretion may be congenital or it may occur suddenly or slowly at any time during life. Most often it may result from pituitary tumor that destroy the pituitary gland. In this condition there is complete alopecia except for the head and tuft of hairs on the legs. In dog showing panhypopituitarism have body weight half the normal size. There is progressive hyper-pigmentation of skin. Permanent dentition is delayed or completely absent in GH deficient dogs. Animals with panhypopituitary dwarfism don't pass through puberty. In male penis and testes remains small in size and in female estrus is irregular or absent.

35. What are the functions of gonadotropins?

Ans. Gonadotrpins include **follicle stimulating hormone (FSH) and luteinizing hormone (LH)**. Some times prolactin is also included among gonadotropins because in certain species it stimulate corpus luteum functioning. **LH** and **FSH** are synthesized and secreted by gonadotropes of the anterior pituitary gland. Both in males and females, FSH stimulates the maturation of germ cells. In **males**, FSH stimulates maturation of seminiferous tubule and spermatogenesis. In **females**, FSH initiates follicular growth, specifically affecting granulosa cells. Like LH, FSH release at pituitary gland is controlled by pulses of gonadotropin releasing hormone (GnRH). In females, LH supports thecal cells in the ovary that provide androgens as precursors for estradiol production. LH surge triggers ovulation and development of corpus luteum that in turn, produces progesterone to prepare the endometrium for implantation. In male, LH had also been called interstitial cell stimulating hormone (ICSH) which acts on leydig cells of the testis for the production of testosterone.

36. What is the function of antidiuretic hormone (ADH)?

Ans. **ADH** is otherwise called as **vasopressin**. It increases water reabsorption from distal convoluted tubule and collecting ducts of the kidney. Both DCT and collecting ducts are totally impermeable to water in absence of ADH. ADH cause special structural changes in the membrane of the tubular epithelial cells which provides many temporary new pores that cause free diffusion of water through pores. Large amount of ADH has a potent effect on the blood vessels particularly in arteries. It causes constriction of the arteries in all parts of the body. Due to vasoconstriction the blood pressure is increased. However the amount of ADH required to cause the vasopressure effect is very much more than the amount required to cause antidiuretic effect.

37. What is function of oxytocin?

Ans. **Oxytocin** acts on mammary gland and uterus. On uterus it cause contraction of myoepithelial cells especially towards end of gestation which helps in expulsion of fetus. Oxytocin also facilitates the transport of sperms through female genital tract upto fallopian tube by producing uterine contraction. On mammary gland oxytocin cause ejection of milk from mammary gland. The process by which milk is ejected from alveoli of mammary gland is called **milk ejection reflex**.

38. What is function of prolactin?

Ans. Prolactin regulates lactation. Prolactin stimulates mammary gland to produce milk. It cause enlargement of mammary gland and increases the production of milk. It stimulate proliferation of oligodendrocyte precursor cells. These cells differentiate into oligodendrocytes which are responsible for the formation of myelin coatings on axons in central nervous system. Prolactin also has a number of other effects including contributing to synthesis of the fetal lungs at the end of the pregnancy and immune tolerance of the fetus during pregnancy.

39. What is rickets?

Ans. Rickets occur mainly in children. It results from calcium or phosphate deficiency in the extra cellular fluid caused by lack of vitamin D. If child is exposed adequately to sunlight the 7-dehydrocholesterol in the skin become activated by UV rays and forms vitamin D which prevents rickets by promoting calcium and phosphate absorption from the intestine. Rickets occurs specially in spring. In rickets blood calcium is slightly depressed but the level of phosphate is greatly depressed. This is because parathyroid gland prevents the calcium level falling by promoting bone absorption. During prolonged rickets the marked compensatory increase in PTH secretion causes extreme osteoclastic absorption of the bone. This in turn causes the bone progressively weaker. Supplying of adequate calcium and phosphate in diet and equally important administering large amount of vitamin D is necessary for treatment of rickets. If vitamin D is not administered then little calcium and phosphate are absorbed from the gut.

40. What is osteomalacia or adult rickets?

Ans. Adult seldom have a serious dietary deficiency of vitamin D or calcium because large quantities of calcium are not needed for bone growth like in children. However serious deficiency of both vitamin D and calcium occasionally occurs as a result of steatorrhea (failure to absorb fat) because vitamin D is fat soluble and calcium tend to form insoluble soap with fat. In steatorrhea both vitamin D and calcium tends to pass in to the feces which results osteomalacia and adult rickets develops.

41. What are glucocorticoids?

Ans. Hormones acts on glucose metabolism and hence the name is glucocorticoids. These hormones are mainly secreted by zona faciculata of adrenal cortex. Zona reticularis also secrete a small amount of glucocorticoids. These glucocorticoids include **cortisol** (very potent and constitue 95% of glucocorticoid activity), **corticosterone** (4% of total glucocorticoid activity), **cortisone, prednisone, methyl prednisone** (synthetic and five times potent as cortisol) and **dexamethasone** (synthetic and thirty times potent as cortisol). From these hormones some hormones have both glucocorticoid and mineral corticoid activity. It is also observed that cortisol have small amount of mineral corticoid effects.

42. What are mineral corticoids?

Ans. These hormones acts on the metabolism of the electrolytes or minerals especially sodium and potassium and hence called as mineral corticoids. These hormones are mainly secreted by zona glomerulosa. These mineral corticoids include **aldosterone** (major mineral corticoid and constitute 90% of all mineral corticoids), **deoxy corticosterone** ($1/30^{th}$ as potent as aldosterone), **corticosterone** (slight mineral corticoid activity), **9α-flurocortisol, cortisol, cortisone** etc.

43. What is the effect of aldosterone on sodium and potassium reabsorption?

Ans. Aldosterone acts on the distal convoluted tubule and collecting ducts where it increases the reabsorption of sodium ions and secretion of potassium ions. During hyper secretion of aldosterone the loss of sodium ions through urine is reduced but at the same time loss of potassium in the urine increases several folds. Hyposecretion of aldosteron cause enoromous increase in the loss of sodium ions in the urine and decrease in potassium ions. Therefore aldosterone regulate sodium and potassium ion concentration and osmolarity in the body.

44. What is Cushing syndrome?

Ans. Hyper secretion by the adrenal cortex cause a complex cascade of hormone effects called cushing syndrome. Cushing syndrome is secondary to excess secretion of ACTH which is referred cushing disease. If cushing disease is due to pituitary origin it is called **cushing disease** but if it is adrenal origin it is called **cushing syndrome**. Pituitary origin leads to increase in secretion of ACTH that cause hyperplasia of adrenal cortex leading to excess secretion of glucocorticoids. Adrenal origin cause excess secretion of cortisol that may be due to tumor in zona faciculata of adrenal cortex. In this syndrome there is redistribution of body fat in an abnormal manner from lower part to upper part of abdomen. Face become **moon face.** Extremities of the body become thin. Abdominal wall is stretched and cause rupture of subdermal tissue. Muscle become weak and osteoporosis develops and bone become susceptible to fracture. There is hyperglycemia, glucosuria, hypertension and patient is succeptible to infection because of immunosuppression.

45. What is Conn's syndrome or primary aldosteronism?

Ans. Occasionally a small tumor of zona glomerulosa cell occurs and secrete large amount of aldosterone. This condition is called **primary aldosteronism or conn's syndrome**. Symptom of this condition includes hypokalemia, increase in extra cellular fluid volume, increase in blood volume, increase in sodium ion concentration in blood, there is muscle paralysis due to hypokalemia because low potassium concentration affect transmission of action potential by nerve fiber. There is decrease in plasma renin concentration because of increase in blood pressure due to increase in extra cellular fluid volume.

46. What are Catecholamines and their functions?

Ans. Adrenal medullary hormones combinely called **catecholamines**. There are three types of catecholamines named **adrenaline, nor adrenaline** and **dopamine**.Adrenalin and nor adrenalin exert the same effect as that of sympathetic stimulation. But the effect of hormone is prolonged 10times more than the sympathetic stimulation. This is because inactivation, degredation and removal of these two hormones occurs slowly. The effect of adrenalin or nor adrenalin on various target organs depends upon the types of receptors present in the organ. Adrenalin acts through both α and β receptors equally but noradrenalin acts mostly through β receptors and very slightly through â receptors. Nor adrenalin cause constriction of all the blood vessels of the body, increase activity of heart, inhibit GI tract, dilation of pupil. Adrenalin cause almost the same effects caused by noradrenalin but effects differs in the following respect as i) adrenalin because of its greater effects on â receptors has greater effect on cardiac stimulation than those of nor adrenalin, ii) adrenalin cause weak constriction of blood vessels in muscles where as nor adrenalin cause stronger constriction, iii) nor adrenalin increase blood pressure in greater extend but epinephrine increase blood pressure with lesser extend, iv) adrenalin has 5-10 times greater metabolic effects than noradrenalin v) adrenalin increase metabolic rate 100% above normal that leads to increase in activity and excitability of body.

47. What is the effect of aldosterone on blood pressure?

Ans. Mineral corticoids cause persistent increase in extra cellular fluid and blood volume which finally leads to increase in blood pressure. This increase in blood pressure increases kidney excretion of both salt and water is called pressure natriuresis and pressure dieresis respectively. Thus after extra cellular fluid volume increase 5-15% above normal arterial pressure also increases 15-25mm. This elaveted blood pressure returns the renal output of salt and water to normal despite the excess aldosterone.

48. How corticosteroids shows anti-inflammatory effects?

Ans. Cortisol stabilize the lysosomal membrane because of which proteolytic enzymes stored in lysosome are released slowly. It decreases the permeability of the capillaries due to vasoconstriction because of which there is prevention of blood rush to injured area. Cortisol decreases both migration of WBC into inflamed area and phagocytosis of damaged cells as wel as increases production of RBC. Cortisol lowers fever because it reduces the release of interleukin-1 from WBC which is one of the principal excitants to hypothalamic temperature controlling system. Cortisol also cause resolution of inflammation because immediate effect of cortisol is to block most of the factors that are promoting inflammation but in addition rate of healing is reduced.

Choose the Best Answer

1. Hormones are

a) Chemical regulators that are conveyed from one organ to another via the blood stream
b) Secreted by endocrine cells
c) Secreted by nerve cells
d) a, b and c

2. Most commonly, hormone release is controlled by

a) Positive feedback b) Negative feedback
c) Biofeedback d) Feed forward

3. Intracellular messenger which mediates water soluble hormone action

a) ATP b) CAMP
c) Adenylate cyclase d) None of the above

4. Role of hormones

a) Regulate metabolism b) Stimulate gamete production
c) Control growth d) All of the above

5. An animal fell and was hurt, the anxious feeling that owner felt is caused by

a) Glucagon b) Insulin
c) Epinephrine d) Adrenocorticotropic

6. If one has to take insulin daily, it implies

a) His beta cells don't function correctly
b) His alpha cells don't function correctly
c) His both cells are not functioning correctly
d) His GHRH hormone is not functioning correctly

7. Reason of iodine in salt is to

a) Prevent diabetes
b) Prevent simple goiters
c) Prevent addison's disease
d) Prevent cushing syndrome

8. All hormones react to a negative feedback except

a) Progesterone
b) Estrogen
c) Prolactin
d) Oxytocin

9. If one has a high blood calcium level it may be due to

a) Calcitonin
b) Parathyroid
c) Glucocorticoids
d) Glucagon

10. Hormones that are lipids and are synthesized from cholesterol

a) Protien
b) Amino acid-derived
c) Polypeptide
d) Steroids

11. Hormone must bind to a receptor protein on the plasma membrane of the cell

a) Water soluble
b) Lipid soluble
c) Steroid
d) Polypeptide
e) a and d

12. Endocrine glands release hormones in response to

a) Hormones from other endocrine glands
b) Chemical characteristics of the blood
c) Neural stimulation
d) All of the above

13. Anterior pituitary secretes

a) Oxytocin
b) Endorphins
c) ADH
d) TRH

14. Chief cells produce

a) Epinephrine
b) Glucagon
c) Mineralocoticoids
d) Parathyroid hormone

15. The endocrine system

a) Releases chemicals into the bloodstream for distribution throughout the body
b) Releases hormones that alter the metabolic activities of many tissues and organs
c) Produces effects that can last for hours, days, or even longer
d) Can alter gene activity of cells
e) All of the above

16. Each of the following hormones is an amino acid derivative except

a) Epinephrine
b) Melatonin
c) Thyroxine (T4)
d) Thyroid stimulating hormone (TSH)

17. When adenyl cyclase is activated

a) cAMP is formed
b) cAMP is broken
c) G-proteins bind to cAMP
d) steroid hormones enter the cell

18. Which of the following hormones does not act by a second messenger system

a) Glucagon b) Epinephrine
c) Growth hormone d) Testosterone

19. Hypophyseal structure receives signals from the hypothalamus via the hypophyseal portal vein

a) Follicles b) Adenohypophysis
c) Neurohypophysis d) Pars intermedia

20. Low blood glucose level typically results in the secretion of all of the following except

a) Glucagon b) Thyroxine
c) hGH d) PTH

21. Action of glucocorticoids involves many functions, but only one of the following is a correct one

a) Increases inflammatory responses
b) Decreases lipid hydrolysis
c) Increases glucose levels
d) Retention of electrolytes by kidneys

22. Hormone acts on the intestines and increase calcium absorption

a) Calcitonin b) Calcitriol
c) Thyroxine d) Pancreatic polypeptide

23. Thyroid stimulating hormone (TSH) causes all of the following except

a) Activation of thyroid follicular cells
b) Increase iodide trapping in thyroid follicles
c) Increase thyroglobulin synthesis
d) Increase release of T3 and T4
e) All are correct

24. Pancreatic cells that secrete insulin are the

a) Follicular cells b) Alpha cells
c) Beta cells d) Delta cells

25. General adaptation syndrome (GAS) is activated by the

a) Hypothalamus b) Adrenal gland
c) Pituitary gland d) Thyroid gland

26. If one has to eat sugar which hormone would be expected to secrete at higher levels

a) Insulin b) Epinephrine
c) Glucagon d) Cortisol

27. Somatostatin is secreted by

a) Pancreatic F-cells b) Pancreatic delta cells
c) Zona fasciculata d) Parafollicular cells

28. Hyposecretion of cortisol cause

a) Cretinism b) Diabetes mellitus
c) Addison's disease d) Grave's disease

29. A tumor in the adrenal zona glomerulosa can cause

a) Increased blood sodium levels
b) Increased blood glucose levels
c) Decreased blood calcium levels
d) Increased dehydration

30. Oxytocin is secreted by

a) Adenohypophysis
b) Neurohypophysis
c) Zona glomerulosa
d) Pars intermedia

31. Decrease in insulin hormone receptors on cells can result in

a) Diabetes insipidus
b) Type I diabetes mellitus
c) Type II diabetes mellitus
d) Insulin-dependant diabetes mellitus

32. Vasopressin is otherwise called as

a) Cortisol
b) Epinephrine
c) ADH
d) hGH

33. General adaptation syndrome (GAS) is

a) A mechanism to maintain homeostasis under stress
b) To resets the levels of controlled conditions in the body in response to stress
c) A part of the sympathetic response
d) To reduces the amounts of stress your body encounters

34. Which of the following characteristics is the same for the nervous and endocrine systems

a) Target cells affected
b) Time to onset of actions
c) Duration of actions
d) Mechanism of signalling and communication
e) None of the above

35. The process by which hormones are released from their secretor cells are called

a) Pinocytosis
b) Exocytosis
c) Phapocytosis
d) Enclocytosis

36. The precursor of steroid hormones are

a) Arachidonic acid b) Cholesterol
c) Estradiole d) Pospholipid

37. The receptors of protein hormones are located in

a) Golgi bodies b) Nuclear membrane
c) Cell wall d) Cell membrane

38. Which one of the following is a amino acid derived hormone

a) Progesterone b) ACTH
c) Thyroid d) Estrogen

39. Excess of growth hormone secretion in childhood cause

a) Cushing syndrome b) Gigantism
c) Osteomalasia d) Acromegali

40. Hypertrophy and Hyperplacia is due to influence of which hormone

a) Thyroid b) ACTH
c) Growth hormone d) Steroid hormone

41. Diabetes inspidus is mainly due to decrease of which hormone

a) Insulin b) Thyroid
c) Oxytocin d) ADH

42. Biologically most active form of thyroid hormone is

a) T3 b) T4
c) MIT d) DIT

43. Which one of the following is an autoimmune disease

a) Grave's disease b) Myxedema
c) Cushing syndrome d) Cretinism

44. Hormone that increase the blood calcium level is

a) Calcitonin b) Paratyroid hormone
c) Aldosterone d) Insulin

45. Hormone that control the ECF volme is

a) Aldosterone b) Thyroid
c) ACTH d) MSH

46. Hormone that is called as life saving hormone

a) ADH b) Aldoserone
c) Testosterone d) Estrogen

47. Hormone that is called as life protecting hormone

a) ADH b) Aldoserone
c) Cortisol d) Throid

48. Hormone promoting RBCs production is secreted by

a) Kidney b) Bone marrow
c) Spleen d) Liver

49. Progesterone is mainly secreted from

a) Corpus luteum b) Ovary
c) Placenta d) Uterus

50. Hormone responsible for maturity in male is

a) Progesterone b) Estrogen
c) Testosterone d) All

51. Androgens are secreted by

a) Testes b) Ovary
c) Thyroid gland d) Pituitary gland

52. Spermatogenesis is under the regulation of

a) Vasopressin b) FSH
c) LH d) Testosterone

53. Secretion of androgen by testes is regulated by

a) Oxytocin b) FSH
c) LTH d) ICSH

54. Testosterone is secreted by

a) Sperm b) Seminiferous tubules
c) Leydig cells d) Prostate gland

55. Release of oocytes in mammal occurs mainly under the influence of

a) FSH and LH b) TSH and STH
c) ACTH and GH d) TSH and ACTH

56. Contraceptive pills normally contain

a) Aldosterone b) Progesterone
c) Cortisol d) Testosterone

57. Steroid hormones have a common structure of

a) Cholesterol b) Triglyceride
c) Tyrosine d) Phospholipid

58. Ovulation in mammal is due to sudden surge of which hormone

a) FSH b) LH
c) Progesterone d) Estrogen

59. Ovarian hormones are usually ________ in nature

a) Protein b) Amino acid
c) Fat d) Steroid

60. High level of progesterone in blood suppress the release of

a) LH b) ACTH
c) FSH d) All

61. Hormone which is secreted by kidney is

a) Gastrin b) Aldosterone
c) Seretin d) Erythropoietin

62. Receptors for protein hormone is located at

a) Cytoplasm b) Surface of plasma membrane
c) Nucleus d) Endoplasmic reticulum

63. MSH is secreted from

a) Anterior pituitary b) Posterior pituitary
c) Median lobe of pituitary d) All

64. Temporary endocrine structure after ovulation is

a) Corpus callosum b) Corpus luteum
c) Corpus albicans d) Corpus uteri

65. Hormone that maintains pregnancy is

a) Estrogen b) Oxytocin
c) Relaxin d) Progesterone

66. Corpus luteum mainly secrete hormone

a) Progesterone b) Estrogen
c) FSH d) LH

67. Hormone responsible for BMR is

a) Growth hormone b) Steroids
c) Gonadotropin d) Thyroid hormone

68. Ghrelin is secreted from

a) Stomach b) Brain
c) Both a & b d) Pituitary

69. Leptin is secreted from

a) Stomach b) Brain
c) Adipose tissue d) Pituitary

70. Hormones those are water soluble and don't require carrier proteins for transport are

a) Steroid hormones b) Protein and peptide hormones
c) Both a & b d) Thyroid hormones

71. Hormones those are water insoluble and require carrier proteins for transport are

a) Steroid hormones b) Thyroid hormones
c) Both a & b d) Protein and peptide hormones

72. Hormones whose receptors are present in cell cytoplasm

a) Steroid hormones b) Protein and peptide hormones
c) Thyroid hormones d) All

73. Hormones whose receptors are present in cell nucleus

a) Steroid hormones b) Protein and peptide hormones
c) Thyroid hormones d) All

74. Hormones whose receptors are present on the surface of the cell membrane

a) Steroid hormones b) Protein and peptide hormones
b) Thyroid hormones d) All

75. Hormones that contains 100 amino acids or more are called

a) Peptides b) Protein hormone
c) Steroid hormone d) None

76. The process by which hormone is secreted directly to blood stream is called

a) Endocytosis b) Diapedesis
c) Exocytosis d) Oozing out

77. Hormones that act through adenyl cyclase–cAMP second messenger system is/are

a) ACTH b) LH and FSH
c) HCG d) All

78. Hormones that act through phospholipid second messenger system is/are

a) Oxytocin
b) Thyroid releasing hormone
c) Gonadotropin releasing hormone
d) All

79. Whch gland is called as master gland of body

a) Hypothalamus b) Pituitary
c) Thyroid d) Adrenal

80. Pars intermedia is almost absent in ___________

a) Cattle and buffalo b) Sheep and Goat
c) Human d) Pig

81. Embryologically anterior pituitary is originated from

a) Rathke's pouch
b) Neural tissue out growth of hypothalamus
c) Esophageal diverticulum
d) Invagination of cardia

82. Rathke's pouch is an embryonic invagination of

a) Stomach epithelium b) Pharyngeal epithelium
c) Esophageal epithelium d) Cardiac spithelium

83. Embryologically posterior pituitary is originated from

a) Rathke's pouch
b) Neural tissue out growth of hypothalamus
c) Esophageal diverticulum
d) Invagination of cardia

84. GH exerts much of its effect through an intermediate substance secreted by liver is

a) Somatostatin
b) Somatotropin
c) Somatomedin
d) None

85. Somatomedin is also called as

a) Insulin like growth factor
b) Somatostatin
c) Growth hormone
d) All

86. Half life of IGF I is longer than growth hormone because

a) GH binds loosely with plasma protein
b) GH binds strongly with plasma protein
c) IGF 1 binds loosely with plasma protein
d) IGF 1 binds strongly with plasma protein

87. Peptide secreted from stomach and hypothalamus and stimulate secretion of growth hormone is

a) Ghrelin
b) Leptin
c) Motilin
d) Enterostatin

Answers

1. d	2. b	3. b	4. d	5. c	6. a	7. b	8. d	9. b	10. d
11. e	12. d	13. b	14. d	15. e	16. d	17. a	18. d	19. b	20. d
21. c	22. b	23. e	24. c	25. a	26. a	27. b	28. c	29. a	30. b
31. c	32. c	33. b	34. e	35. b	36. b	37. d	38. c	39. b	40.c
41. d	42. a	43. a	44. b	45. a	46. b	47. c	48. a	49. a	50. c
51. b	52. b	53. d	54. c	55. a	56. b	57. a	58. b	59. d	60. a
61. d	62. b	63. c	64. b	65. d	66. a	67. d	68. c	69. c	70. b
71. c	72. a	73. c	74. b	75. b	76. c	77. d	78. d	79. a	80. c
81. a	82. b	83. b	84. c	85. a	86. d	87.a			

□□□

CHAPTER-5

Reproductive System

Embryogenically male genital system/organs are originated from **mesohephric duct or wolfian duct** where as female genital systems are formed from **paramesonephric duct or mullerian duct.** The main functional parts of male genital system of domestic animals are penis, scrotum, testes, rete testes, efferent tubules, epididymis, vasa deferentia and accessory glands like prostate, seminal vesicles and bulbourethral glands. Female reproductive organs are composed of ovaries, oviduct, uterus, cervix, vagina and valva.

Histologically each **testes** is composed of several crypts enclosed in a serous layer called Tunica Vaginalis/Albugenia. Each crypt in turn has number of seminiferous tubules. The wall of the seminiferous tubules consists of a basement membrane multilayered sperm producing epithellium having two or three types of cells as **germ cell** ares spermatozoa, **sertoli cell** called sperm mother cell or produce spermatozoa and **leydig cell** which is present in the space between seminiferous tubules and produce male hormones testosterone. For effective function of testes the testes must be maintained at a temperature 2-3°C lower than that of body temperature. Testes secretes several male sex hormones which are collectively called androgens including testosterone, dihydrotestosterone and androstenedione. Tube arising from the dorsal part of testes from the efferent duct consists of three parts as the caput (head) epididymis, corpus (body) and cauda (Tail). The tail of the epididymis leads into vas deferens which is a slender tube. Epididymis has 4 major functions as i) Transport of sperms from rete-testes to efferent duct ii) Cocentration of sperm iii) Maturation of sperm and iv) Storage of sperm. **Urethra** is the common passage for the products of testes, accessory glands and for the excretion of urine. **Accessory glands** provide bulk of their secretion into the urethra at the time of ejaculation. There are 3 types of accessory glands as i) **Seminal vesicles**: these are pair and lies laterally to the terminal part of each ductus deferens. The secretion of seminal vesicles contains high level of **fructose and citric acid** ii) **Prostate gland** whose secretion contain high mineral and iii) **Bulbourethral or Cowper's gland:** These are dorsal to urethra near the termination of its pelvis portion and contribute gel like component of the boar semen. **Penis** is the organ for copulation and composed of erectile tissue. The series of cellular division including the proliferation of spermatogonia and meiotic division is called **spermatocytogenesis**. The halploid cell resulting from this process called **spermatid**. The spermatid then undergoes a progressive series of structural and developmental changes to form spermatozoa. This metamorphic changes called **spermiogenesis.** During embryonic development primordial germ cell divide several times (mitosis) and form cell called **gonocyte**. The round spermatid are transformed into spermatozoa by series of progressive morphologic changes collectively called **spermatogenesis.** The various stages of spermatid transformation are divided into 4 stages as i) Golgi phase ii) Cap phase iii)Acrosomal phase iv) Maturation phase. The final release of formed germ cells into the lumen of the seminiferous tubules is called spermiation. **Cryptorchidism** means failure of testes to descent from abdomen to scrotum at or near the time of birth of fetus.

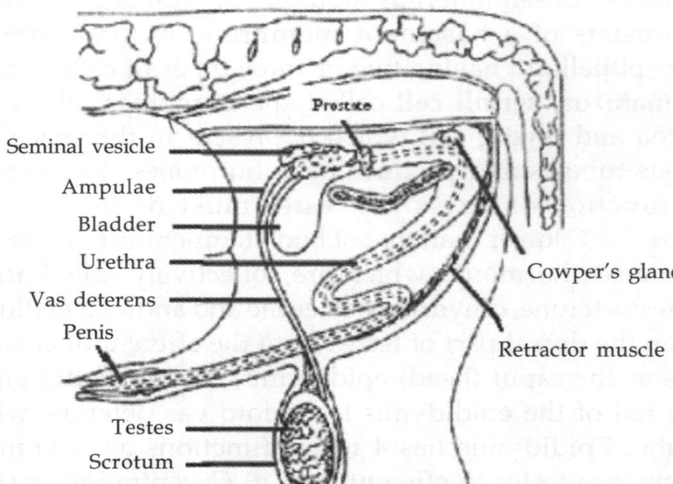

Male reproductive organs (bovine)

Ovary is present in the abdomen and perform both exocrine and endocrine function. Ovary is surrounded by germinal epithelium. Shape of ovary varies from species to species as in cattle and sheep: ovary is almond shape, Horse: ovary is bean shape with ovulation fossae and in pig: ovary looks like cluster of grapes. Ovary is composed of medulla and cortex. **Ovarian cortex** contains several primary follicles and few large follicles. During each oestens cycle variable number of follicles undergo rapid growth and development, culminating in the process of ovulation. The number of graffian follicles that develop per estrus cycle depends on heredity and environmental factors. Both the rate of follicular development and the number that ripen per estrus depends on the pituitary gonadotropins. In cattle and horse one follicle usually develop more rapidly than others so that at each estrus only one egg is released. **Ovarian medulla** consists of loose connective tissue that contains nerve lympatics, tortuous thin walled blood vessels, collogen, elastic fibres, fibroblasts and scattered smooth muscle cells. **Uterus** consists of 2 uterine horn, a body and a neck. The shape of uterus varies from species to species as in cow it is **bipartite** type, in swine it is **bicornuate** type and in sheep and horse it is bipartite. **Cervix** is a sphincter like structure that projects caudally into vagina.

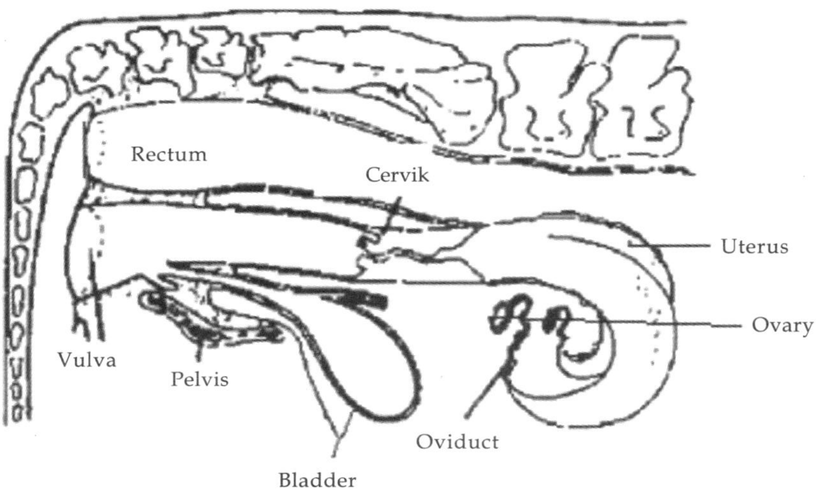

Female reproductive organs (bovine)

Synthesis of Estrogen and Progesterone in testes and ovary is called **steroidogenesis. Estrogen** is mainly required for psychologic manifestation of estrus and development of secondary sexual characteristics in female, glandular duct development of the uterine endometrium and also helps in duct growth in mammary gland during lactogenesis. Where as **progesterone** is always works synergistically with estrogen in several physiologic functions including growth of uterine and mammary gland and it inhibit uterine contractions and stimulate endometrial glands to secrete endometrial fluid which is necessary for nourishment of pre-implantation of blastocyte as well as maintenance of pregnancy. **Puberty** is basically the result of gradual adjustment between increasing gonadotropin activity and the ability of the gonads to simultaneously assume steroidogenesis and gametogenesis. Age of puberty varies with species. It is 12 months in cattle, 15-18 months in horse and 6-7 months in sheep and goat. The **estrus cycle** refers to the rhythmic phenomena observed in all mammals (except in some primates) in which there is regular but limited period of sexual receptivity. Estrus cycle varies from species to species as cow/sow/goat-20-21 days, ewe-16-17 days and mare-20-24 days. Basic system that control the ovarian activity include pulsaile release of gonadotropins from anterior pituitary. Including this factor other factors that modify normal reproductive activity are photoperiod, temperature, social factor and pheromones.

In many species ovulation occurs spontaneously after normal follicle grow during estrus or menstrual cycle. These animals are called **spontaneous ovulation** which include animals like bitch, cow, goat, mare, sow, primates, with laboratory species like rat, mouse and gunea pig. But some animals don't ovulate spontaneously but they need copulation for ovulation. These animals are called **induced ovulators** which include animals like cat, rabbit, camel etc.

Fertilization is the fusion of two gametes to form one cell called zygote. It is other wise defined as period from penetration of sperm to first cleavage. Fertilization is a dual process as i) **embryologic aspect** that involves the activation of ovum by sperm and ii) **genetic aspect** that involves introduction of hereditary materials from sire to ovum. The essential hereditary material is the acrosomal DNA in the sperm nucleus. Maintenance of corpus luteum is essential for establishment of pregnancy in all farm animals. In farm animals the presence of embryo must be signaled before implantation begins to prevent the regression of corpus luteum. The critical period for signaling by the conceptus to block luteolysis and allow pregnancy to establish is called **maternal recognition of pregnancy.** In cow maternal recognition of pregnancy occurs between day 16 to 19 of pregnancy. The bovine conceptus produces number of low molecular weight acidic proteins which include bovine **trophoblast protein-1 (btp-1) called IFN-z.**

Interval from fertile mating to parturition is called **gestation or pregnancy.** Different species have different gestation period. Example: cattle (278 days), buffalo (310 days), sheep (148 days) and goat (150 days). Physiological process by which the pregnant uterus delivers the fetus and placenta from the maternal environment is called **parturition or labor.**

Short Questions and Answers

1. What is wolfian duct and mullerian duct?

Ans. Embryogenically male genital system/organs are originated from **mesohephric duct or wolfian duct** where as female genital systems are formed from **paramesonephric duct or mullerian duct.** Mesonephric duct form epididymis, ductus deferens, vescicular gland and penis where as mullerian duct developed uterus and vagina. Fetal androgen causes development of male reproductive tract. **Mullerian inhibiting substance** a glycoprotein is responsible for suppression of mullerian duct.

2. What is the function of testes?

Ans. Male gonad, called testes having 2 major functions as production of **germ cells** called spermatozoa and production of a**ndrogen** which give the individual male characteristics.

3. What is the function of epididymis?

Ans. Epididymis has 4 major functions as i) Transport: sperms are transported from rete-testes to efferent duct. It takes about 7 to 9 days for any sperm to travel from germinal epithelium to cauda, ii) Cocentration of sperm, iii) Maturation of sperm and iv) Storage of sperm.

4. What are different types of accessory glands and their action?

Ans. Accessory glands provide bulk of their secretion into the urethra at the time of ejaculation. This is rich in carbohydrate, salts, proteins, amino acids, enzymes, vitamins and having relatively high buffer capacity. There are 3 types of accessory glands as

i) **Seminal vesicles:** These are pair and lies laterally to the terminal part of each ductus deferens. The secretion of seminal vesicles contains high level of **fructose and citric acid**. In boar this is large and less compact. In stallion they are large pyriform glandular sac. The duct of seminal vesicle and ductus deferens share a common ejaculating duct that opens to urethra.

ii) **Prostate gland:** The body of prostate is small in bull and large in boar. In stallion it is wholly external. Prostate secretion contain high mineral.

iii) **Bulbourethral or Cowper's gland:** It is paired, round, compact bodies of size of a walnut in the bull. They are large in boar and contribute gel like component of the boar semen.

Function of Accessory glands

i) Liquid vehicle for the transport of sperm, ii) Fructose and citric acid are important component o seminal vesicle secretion of domestic species and iii) Citric acid alone is found in stallion seminal vesicle. Boar seminal vesicle contain little fructose and are characterized by high content of ergothianine and inositol.

5. What is blood testes barrier?

Ans. The seminiferous tubules are not penetrated by blood vessels or lymph vessels. So the germ cells developed within tubules are protected from chemical changes in blood by a specialized permeability barrier called **blood testes barrier**. This barrier mainly formed by serolli cells. This blood testes barrier has mainly two functions as i) Allows the creation of an environment in which the metabolism of spermatozoa is controlled, ii) This protects against the movement of spermatozoa into interstitium of testes.

6. What is spermatogenesis?

Ans. Spermatogenesis is the entire developmental process involves in the transformation of the stem cell or spermatogenium into a spermatozoa in the seminiferous tubules. The seminiferous tubules is composed of 2 basic cell types (i) Sertoli cells (ii) Germ cell. The germ cell undergoes a continuous series of cellular division and developmental changes beginning at the periphery and progressing towards the lumen of tubules. The stem cell called spermatogonia divide several times before forming spermatocyte. The spermatocyte then undergoes meiosis thereby reducing DNA content of the cell to half. The series of cellular division including the proliferation of spermatogonia and meiotic division is called **spermatocytogenesis**. The halploid cell resulting from this process called **spermatid**. The spermatid then undergoes a progressive series of structural and developmental changes to form spermatozoa. This metamorphic changes called **spermiogenesis.**

7. What is spermatocytogenesis?

Ans. During embryonic development primordial germ cell divide several times (mitosis) and form cell called **gonocyte**. These gonocyte undergo differentiation and form AO **spermatogonia**, which followed by formation of A1, A2, A3, A4 spermatogonia. The A4 spermatogonia divide again o form **intermediate spermatogonia**. This intermediate then form **B-spermatogonia**. The B-spermatogonia form **primary spermatocyte**. Upto this stage of development there is mitosis. After initial mitosis there are 4 mitosis in Bull, Buck (rabbit) and Ram. 5 mitosis in rat and 3 mitosis in man. Primary spermatocyte undergo meiotic division to form secondary spermatocyte .Though the cells are haploid but a further division is required to form **spermatid**.

8. What is spermiogenesis?

Ans. The round spermatid are transformed into spermatozoa by series of progressive morphologic changes collectively called **spermatogenesis.** These changes include condensation of nuclear chromatin formation of sperm tail and development of acrosomal cap.

The various stages of spermatid transformation are divided into 4 stages

A) Golgi phase B) Cap phase C) Acrosomal phase D) Maturation phase

A) Golgi phase

This stage is characterized by

i) Formation of proacrosomal granules within the golgi apparatus.

ii) Coalescence of the granules into a single acrosomal granule

iii) Adherence of acrosomal granules to the nuclear envelop

iv) Early stage of tail development

B) Cap phase

This stage is characterized by

i) Spreading of adherent acrosomal granules over the surface of the spermatic nucleus

ii) This process continuous until 2/3 rd of the anterior portion of the spermatid nucleus is covered by thin, double layered membranous sac that closely adhere to the nuclear envelop.

iii) Development of axonomal component of tail

C) Acrosonal phase

This stage is characterized by

i) Major changes in nuclei, acrosome and tail

ii) Nuclear changes include condensation of chromatin into dense granule

iii) Reshaping of the spheroidal nucleus into an elongated, flattened structure

iv) Acrosome condenses and elongates to the corresponded to the shape of nucleus

v) The changes in nuclear morphology are accompanied by displacement of the cytoplasm to the caudal aspect of the nucleus where it surrounds the portion of the developing tail

vi) Mitochondria which were distributed throughout the cytoplasm of the spermatid begin to concentrate close to the axoneme where they form the sheath that characterize the middle piece of the tail.

D) Maturation phase

This stage is characterized by

i) Final transformation of the elongated spermatid to be released into the lumen of the seminiferous tubules

ii) Reshaping of the nucleus and acrosome of each spermatid

iii) Within nucleus the chromatin granules undergo progressive condensation as the transitional proteins

iv) There is formation of fibrous sheath and underlying nine coarse fibers are formed around axoneme.

9. What is spermiation?

Ans. The release of formed germ cells into the lumen of the seminiferous tubules is called **spermiation**. The elongated spermatids which are oriented perpendicularly to the tubular wall are gradually extruded into the lumens of the tubule.

10. What is spermatogenic wave?

Ans. The stages of the cycle of seminiferous epithelium changes not only with time but also along the length of the tubular loop. The sequential changes in a stage of cycle along the length of the tubule in called wave of the seminiferous epithelium/spermatogenic wave.

11. What is chemical composition of spermatozoa?

Ans. Principal composition of spermatozoa is nucleic, acid, proteins and lipids. Nearly 1/3 rd of dry weight of single sperm cell is contributed by nucleus. The nuclear chromatin is composed of approximately half DNA and half protein. Spermatozoa is highly in phosphorous, nitrogen and sulphur.

12. What is male sex hormones?

Ans. Testes secretes several male sex hormones which are collectively called **androgens** including testosterone, dihydrotestosterone and androstenedione. Testosterone is abundant than others and can consider it to be the significant testicular hormone. Testosterone is formed by the interstitial cells of leydig which lies in the interstices between the seminiferous tubules. Leydig cells are almost nonexistent in the testes during childhood when testes secretes almost no testosterone, but they are numerous in the newborn male for the first few months of life and in the adult male any time after puberty. When there is tumour in leydig cells, testosterone secretion increases profusely.

13. What is function of testosterone?

Ans. Testosterone stimulate late stages of spermatogenesis and prolong the span of epididymal sperm, promote growth, development and secretory activity of accessory sex organs of male, maintain secondary sex characteristics and sexual behavior or libido of the male, testosterone is responsible for distinguishing characteristics of masculine body and cause descent of testes into scrotum, after puberty, the increasing amount of testosterone secretion cause penis, scrotum and testes to enlarge, testosterone causes baldness as of production of large quantity of testosterone and cause typical adult masculine voice, increases the thickness of skin and increases the rate of secretion of sebaceous gland, increases protein formation and muscle development, increases bone matrix, so bone grows considerably thicker and strength so testosterone is used in older men to treat osteoporosis, testosterone increases basal metabolism by 15% and increases RBC/cubic mm by 15–20%.

14. What is cryptorchidism?

Ans. Cryptorchidism means failure of testes to descent from abdomen to scrotum at or near the time of birth of fetus. During the development of male fetus, the testes are derived from the **genital** ridge in the abdomen. After that the testes normally descent through inguinal canal into the scrotum. Occasionally this descent doesn't occur or occurs incompletely, so that one or both the testes remains in the abdomen. Testes that remains throughout life in the abdominal cavity is incapable of forming sperm operation to relocate the cryptorchid testes from abdominal cavity into the scrotum before the beginning of adult sexual life are frequently performed who have undescended testes. Testosterone secretion by fetal testes themselves in the normal stimulus cause the testes to descend into the scrotum from abdomen. So instances of cryptorchidism are caused by abnormally formed testes that are unable to secrete enough testosterone.

15. Ovary is which type of gland exocrine or endocrine?

Ans. Ovary is present in the abdomen and perform both exocrine and endocrine function. Exocrine action is by egg release and endocrine action is by hormone synthesis.

16. What are the types of follicles in the ovary?

Ans: There are different types of follicle as per their development in ovary

i) **Primordial follicle**–Oocyte surrounded by 1 layer of flattened follicular cells

ii) **Primary follicle**–Oocyte enclosed by 2–3 layers of cuboidal follicular cells

iii) **Secondary follicle**–Oocye with increase in diameter or number of follicular cells layer with zona pellucida.

iv) **Tertiary follicle**–Here there is secretion of fluid by granulose cells of multilayered follicle by the influence of gonadotropin which accumulate in intercellular spaces formed Antrum. Here zona pellucida surrounded by a solid mass of radiating follicular cells forming corona radiate.

v) **Graffian follicle**–Here follicular cells increase in size, antrum filled with follicular fluid, oocyte pressed at one side surrounded by accumulation of follicular cells called cumulus oophorus. Membrana granulose is formed in this follicle.

vi) **Preovulatory follicle**–Blister like structure protruding from ovarian surface due to rapid accumulation of follicular fluid. Here there is thining of granulosa cell layer and Formation of zona pellucida. There is extrusion of first polar body.

17. How many number of follicles that develop per estrus cycle?

Ans. The number of graffian follicles that develop per estrus cycle depends on heredity and environmental factors. In cattle and horse one follicle usually develop more rapidly than others so that at each estrus only one egg is released. The remaining follicle then regress and become atrophied. In swine 10–25 follicles ripen at each estrus. In Sheep 1–3 follicles reach to maturity. Caloric intake also influence ovulation rate.

18. What is the hormonal mechanism of follicular development?

Ans. Both the rate of follicular development and the number that ripen per estrus depends on the pituitary gonadotropins. Growing follicle is always influenced by FSH from pituitary gland, which helps follicle to undergo growth and maturation. Steroidogenesis by granlosa cells is unique feature of follicular development. Estrogen are generated by theca cells of follicle whereas progesterone is produced by granulosa cells. Following ovulation the granulosa cells are vascularised and secrete increased amount of progesterone.

19. What is follicular fluid?

Ans. It is transudate of blood plasma which provides suitable environment for developing oocyte. This fluid plays a role in differentiation and steroidogenic capacity of ovarian cells. Follicular fluid exerts several effects on spermatozoa such as stimulation of sperm respiration, increased rate of motility and amplitude of flagellar beat and alteration in the acrosome.

20. What is ovulation and its mechanism?

Ans. At ovulation, the egg is released while embedded in a solid mass of follicular cells called **cumules oophrous** which protrudes into the fluid filled **antrum**. The cumulus is usually attached to the granulosa cells opposite the side that will eventually rupture. This rupture occurs at the apex of the follicle. The outermost layer is the first to part. Then there is gradual thining on the surface of the ovary and becomes completely avascular and finally rupture the oocyte called ovulation. Ovulation occurs in response to a LH surge. This preovulatory release of LH causes increased prostaglandin (PGF) synthesis in the ovary leading to increased steroidogenesis and ovulation.

21. What are the functions of uterus?

Ans. i) It helps in transportation of sperm transport from the site of ejaculation to the site of fertilization.

ii) Regulate the function corpus luteum.

iii) Initiation of implantation, pregnancy and parturition.

22. What are the functions of cervix?

Ans. i) It facilitates sperm transport through cervical mucus to the uterine lumen.

ii) It acts as sperm reservoir .Thus release subsequently.

iii) It may play a role in the selection of viable sperm, thus preventing the transport of non viable and defective sperm.

23. What are the functions of vagina?

Ans. i) It is a copulatory organ in which semen is deposited.

ii) Vagina contains no gland. Its walls are moistened by transudates through he vaginal epithelium by cervical mucus and by endometrial secretion.

iii) The pH of vaginal secretion is unfavorable to sperm. A complex interaction of cervical mucus, vaginal secretion and seminal plasma induces a buffering system that protects sperm until they are transported through the micelles of cervical mucus.

iv) Vagina serves as an excretory duct for secretion of cervix, endometrium and oviduct.

iv) It serves as the birth canal during partuirition.

24. What is steroidogenesis?

Ans. Synthesis of Estrogen and Progesterone is called **steroidogenesis.** The immediate precursor of all steroids are pregnenolone which is derived from cholesterol. Pregnenolone subsequently converted to progesterone. Progesterone is converted to testosterone and finally estrogen is produced from testosterone by aromatization.

25. What is function of estrogen?

Ans. i) Required for psychologic manifestation of estrus and development of secondary sexual characteristics in female.

ii) Glandular duct development of the uterine endometrium.

iii) Histological changes in vaginal epithelium during estrus period.

iv) Estrogen helps in duct growth in mammary gland during lactogenesis.

v) Estrogen potentiate the effect of oxytocin and prostaglandins on uterine contraction.

vi) Estrogen assist in the process of implantation.

vii) Non reproductive effects of estrogen include stimulation of calcium uptake and ossification of bones.

viii) Estrogen increases body weight gain by anabolic effect.

ix) Subterranean clover and alfalfa are plant estrogen.

x) Estrogen exert both positive and negative feedback control on LH and FSH release through hypothalamus.

xi) DESC (Diethylstilbasterol) is synthetic non steroidal estrogen. It acts with estrogen receptor and acts with same potency as estrogen.

xii) In cow and sheep estrogen has luteolytic property (CL Regress) where as in sow estrogen has lueotrophic action (maintain CL).

26. What is function of progesterone?

Ans. i) Progesterone always works synergestically with estrogen in several physiologic functions including growth of uterine and mammary gland.

ii) Progesterone inhibit uterine contractions and stimulate endometrial glands to secrete endometrial fluid which is necessary for nourishment of pre-implantation of blastocyte.

iii) Progesterone is responsible for maintenance of pregnancy.

iv) High level of progesterone inhibit estrus and ovulatory surge of LH which prevents ovulation used in birth control pills.

v) Progesterone develop secretory tissue (alveoli) of mammary gland.

vi) Progesterone inhibit uterine motility

vii) Clinically Progesterone is given to prevent abortion in females who are prone to abortion as of sufficient secretion of endogenous progesterone.

27. What is puberty?

Ans. A male or female reached to puberty when it is able to release gametes and to manifest complete sexual behavior sequences. Puberty is basically the result of gradual adjustment between increasing gonadotropin activity and the ability of the gonads to simultaneously assume steroidogenesis and gametogenesis. At the onset of puberty the gonadotropin concentration increases both in amplitude and frequency. In male in response to gonadotropin secretion testosterone progressively rises from very low level to adult level. Age of puberty is influenced by physical environment, photo period, age, breed of dam, breed of sire, environmental temperature, body weight, nutrition. Dairy cattle reach puberty when the body weigh is 30-40% of adult body weight, where as in beef cattle this body weight is abou45-55%.

Age of puberty of different animals

Animals	**Age of puberty**
Rabbit	3-4 months
Sheep/Goat/Swine	6-7 months
Cattle	12 months
Horse	15-18 months

28. What is estrus cycle?

Ans. Estrus is derived from a greek word oistros means gadfly which describes the behavior of cows when attacked by such flies. In non primate mammals, female mating behavior is limited to the estrus period around ovulation. Genetically two types of reproductive cycles are recognized as estrual and menstrual. The estrus cycle refers to the rhythmic phenomena observed in all mammals (except in some primates) in which there is regular but limited period of sexual receptivity. Estrus cycle varies from species to species as Ewe-16-17 days, Mare-20-24 days, Cow/Sow/Goat-20-21 days. Times of ovulation also varies from species to species Ewe-30-36 hr from beginning of estrus, Cow-10-11 hr after end of estrus, Mare-1-2 days before end of estrus, Sow-35-45 hr from beginning of estrus, Goat-30-36 from beginning of estrus.

Esrus cycle is of 4 stages as

i) **Estrus**-It is the time of sexual receptivity, with ovulation usually occurring about the end of esrus.

ii) **Metestrus**-It is the period of early Corpus luteum development. The onset is usually defined as beginning with the end of estrus.

iii) **Diestrus**-It is the period of mature luteal activity that begins about 4 days after ovulation and ends with the regression of CL. Here CL is functional. It is the longest phase of cycle.

iv) **Proestrus**-It is the period of rapid follicle growth that preceeds he onset of estrus. In large domestic species this phase occurs after regression of CL.

One **cycle interval** is defined as the time from the onset of one period of sexual receptivity to the next or the interval between successive ovulation.

29. What is pheromones and its example?

Ans. It is the chemical compound that allows the communication between animals of same species. Pheromones are important for modifying the behavior of both males and females. Males are attracted to females by odors emit from vaginal secretion.

Methyl-P-hydroxy benzoate is an example of pheromone secreted from dog vagina. Females are also influenced by odor of male. Boar urine contain 5á-androsterone. There are different classic phenomena has been reported in mice. The **Whitten effect** which involves the synchronization of estrus cycle by the introduction of male in to group of female. Another example of pheromone is **Bruce effect** which involves the manipulation of pregnancy by pheromones. If a recently bred female mouse is placed in a cage with a strange male, the pregnancy fails. This is due to blockage of prolactin secretion and decline in prolactin cause CL regression and pregnancy fails. Same pheromone effect has already been detected in sheep which is called **Ram effect** which involves in synchronization of estrus if there is introduction of ram into a breeding block of sheep.

30. What is difference between estrus and menstrual cycle?

Ans. There is loss of endometrial epithelium during estrus where as there is estrogen mediated capillary fragility in the endometrium as of which there is bleeding during menstrual cycle in primates.

31. What is folliculogenesis?

Ans. Primordial follicle formed during fetal life or soon after birth some primordial follicle began to grow continuously throughout life or at least until the reserve is exhausted. This grow until ovulation or until the follicle degenerates. The largest follicle is responsible for most estrogen secretion by the ovary at estrus. Estrogen secretion by the largest follicle decreases rapidly at the time of LH peak. The growth of follicle **upto stage at antrum formation is not gonadotropin dependent**. So antrum formation and ovulation are entirely FSH and LH dependent. FSH plays major role in Antrum formation. This FSH stimulates granulose cell mitosis and follicular fluid formation. Estrogen enhances mitotic effect of FSH. On the other hand theca cells are stimulated by LH.

32. What is mechanism of ovulation?

Ans. Ovulation occur in response to several physiologic, Biochemical and Biological mechanism.

Biochemical mechanism of ovulation

The pre ovulatory surge of gonadotropin first induces an immediate and temporary rise in steroid level due to increase in secretion of progesterone. Later estrogen and prostaglandin also augmented. Thus gonadotropin surge induess ovulation by cascade of biochemical changes. Prostaglandin play a basic role in follicular rupture. Inhibition of their sysnthesis always prevent ovulation.

Neuromuscular mechanism of ovulaion

The ovarian stroma and concentric layers of the theca externa of preovulatory follicle contain smooth muscle cells that are richly inervated by autonomic nerve terminal. The frequency of ovarian contraction begins to increase two to three hours before ovulation. This contraction is facilitated by PGF2 leads to follicular rupture. After ovulation the oocyte is picked up by the mucosal fold of the fimbria of oviduct.

33. What is spontanity of ovulation?

Ans. In many species ovulation occurs spontaneously after normal follicle grow during estrus or menstrual cycle. This means a secretory pattern of estrogen is associated with developing dominant follicle with surge of LH is needed for ovulation. This is called **spontaneous ovulation**. Example-bitch, cow, goat, mare, sow, primates, with laboratory species like rat, mouse and gunea pig. But some animals don't ovulate spontaneously but they need copulation for ovulation. These animals are called **induced ovulators** which include animals like cat, rabbit, camel etc. In these animals due to vaginal stimulus there is release of LH through sensory pathway in spinal cord.

34. What is fertilization?

Ans. It is the fusion of two gamets to form one cell called zygote. It is other wise defined as period from penetration of sperm to first cleavage. **Fertilization is a dual process as embryologic aspect and genetic aspect. Embryologic aspect** involves the activation of ovum by sperm. Without the stimulus of fertilization the ovum does not begins to cleave and no embryologic development occurs. **Genetic aspect** include fertilization that involves the introduction of hereditary materials from sire to ovum. The essential hereditary material is the acrosomal DNA in the sperm nucleus. Fusion of male and female gamete is called syngamy is thought as the central process of fertilization. In most of the mammalian species site of fertilization is ampullary isthmus junction. **Fertilization includes the events like** ovum maturation, sperm maturation (capacitation and acrosomal reaction), penetration of sperm to oocyte, block of polyspermy, cortical granule reaction, development of male and female pro nuclei, fusion and cleavage.

35. What is capacitation and acrosomal reaction?

Ans. **Capacitation** of sperm occurs in uterus specially in the isthmus region of the oviduct. Here sperm surface components like cholesterol is removed and there is alteration in glycominoglycans. In other words capacitation is the rubbing sperm surface adsorved materials (including seminal plasma proteins) against cervical mucus. During this capacitation the sperm surface phospholipids bilayer is destabilized and leads to **acrosomal reaction**. The true acrosomal reaction involves the fusion of sperm plasma membrane with the outer acrosomal membrane followed by vesiculation over the anterior segment of the acrosome. During this acrosomal reaction there is massive influx of calcium ions. Fusion and vesiculation of the acrosome released enzymes like hylarunidase and acrosin which helps in penetration of sperm to oocyte.

36. What is implantation?

Ans. In ruminants conceptus attachment involves both caruncular and inner caruncular areas of the uterine endometrium. Growth of the caruncles are stimulated by progesterone. Following implantation there is formation of amnion and allantois. Amnion forms over the embryo. The yolk sac regresses during 2nd to 3rd week of pregnancy as the allantois expands to fuse with chorion.

37. What is maternal recognition of pregnancy?

Ans. Maintenance of CL is essential for establishment of pregnancy in all farm animals. The conceptus synthesizes and secrete seroids and proteins in order to signal its presence to the maternal system and block the regression of CL. In farm animals the presence of embryo must be signaled before implantation begins to prevent the regression of CL. The critical period for signaling by the conceptus to block luteolysis and allow pregnancy to establish is called **maternal recognition of pregnancy.** In cow maternal recognition of pregnancy occurs between day 16 to 19 of pregnancy. The bovine conceptus produces number of low molecular weight acidic proteins which include bovine **trophoblast protein-1 (btp-1) called IFN-ζ.**

38. What are changes in reproductive organs during pregnancy?

Ans. **Vulva and Vagina:** The vulva become edematous and vascular. The vaginal mucosa is pale and dry during most of gestation but is edematous and pliable towards the end of pregnancy.

Cervix: During gestation, the developing fetus is retained within the uterus by tight closure of the external os of the cervix. Highly viscid mucus seals the cervical canal. This so called mucous plug of pregnancy is liquefies and discharged immediately before parturition.

Uterus: As pregnancy progress, the uterus undergoes gradual enlargement to accommodate the growing fetus. The mechanism that permit the enormous increase in size are unknown but are probably hormonals.

Ovary: During pregnancy Cl persists as CL verum as a result estrus cycle is suspended.

Pelvic ligament: Relaxation of the pelvic ligaments occurs gradually during course of pregnancy but becomes more rapid with approaching of parturition.

39. Hormones of pregnancy?

Ans. **Progesterone:** It is key hormone necessary for maintenance of pregnancy. The CL persists through out the pregnancy in all farm animals except in horse. The source of Progesterone during later half of pregnancy is from placenta in mare and ewe and from CL in cow, sow and goat.

Estrogen: There is species difference in urinary excretion of estrogen. In mare estrogen concentration remains low during first 3 months pregnancy, then rise steadily to reach a peak between 9th and 11th month there after decline rapidly to term. In cow maximum excresion of estrogen occurs at 9 months of pregnancy.

Chorionic Gonadotropin: Between 40-130 days of gestation high concentration of equine chorionic gonadotropin also called PMSG are present in maternal blood or urine not in fetal blood. This is secreted by trphoblast cell. This hormone is used to detect pregnancy.

40. What is placenta and its types?

Ans. A unique feature of mammalian development is the provision of nutrients from maternal system by the way of placenta. The **placenta** is an apposition or fusion of the fetal membrane to the endometrium to permit physiologic exchange between fetus and mother. The size and function of placenta changes continuously during the course of pregnancy and eventually expelled. The morphogenesis of the placenta during early gestation is closely related to fetal membrane that are differentiated into yolk sac, amnion , allantois and chorion. The fetal membrane participate in the formation of placenta either separately or in certain combination like chorionic, chorioallantois and yolk sac placentation. Among these chorioallntois placentation in the characteristic of all farm animals. The chorioallantois placenta is classified according to gross shape, microscopic characteristic of maternal fetal barrier and loss of maternal tissue at birth.

41. What is parturition?

Ans. It is the physiological process by which the pregnant uterus delivers the fetus and placenta from the maternal environment.

Sign of parturition

i) Enlargement and edema of vulva

ii) Teat of mammary gland become swollen and secretion through the teat orifice

iii) Nest building is a feature of pig

iv) Cattle and sheep seek isolation from herd just before the onset of parturition.

42. What is mechanism of parturition?

Ans. Parturition is triggered by the fetus and is completed by a complex interaction of endocrine, neural and mechanical factors. Both **fetal** and **maternal** mechanism plays role in initiating of partuiritition.

Fetal mechanism

A significant increase in fetal plasma concentration of cortisol occurs during final stage of gestation as of which there is decrease in fetal progesterone concentration that cause dilatation of cervix. A similar mechanism involving the activation of fetal pituitary adrenal axix which is activated by placentl production prostaglandin E2 leading to rise in fetl cortisol. This fetal cortisol induces the enzyme to catalyse the conversion of progesterone to estrogen. The elevated level of estrogen simulate the secretion of prostaglandin and oxytocin. During the process of parturition progesterone blocks myometrial contraction but as of decrease in progesterone concentration and increase in estrogen concentration at the time of parturition overcomes the progesterone blocks of myometrial contraction and there is increase in spontaneous myometrial contraction. Simultaneously release of oxytocin and prostaglandin stimulate myometrial contraction which cause parturition.

Maternal mechanism

Maternal contribution is less dynamic than fetus. Fetus determines the day of parturition where s mother decides the hour of parturition. Changes in maternal plasma concentration of progesterone and estrogen is associated with parturition. Anxiety, stress or fear prolongs the act of parturition as of decrease in myometrial contraction due to release of epinephrine. Feeding also influence the time of parturition.

43. What is Labor?

Ans. It commences with the onset of regular, peristaltic uterine contraction accompanied by progressive dilatation of the cervix. There are 3 stages of labor **dilation of cervix, expulsion of fetus** and **expulsion of fetal membrane**

Expulsion of the fetus is the shortest of the 3 stages. Labor requires large amount of mechanical energy which is provided mainly by the myometrium and leads to cervical dilation, vaginal stretch and distention and delivery of fetus. The distention of cervix and vagina by conceptus initiates a reflex called Ferguson's reflex which produces the expulsive forces of abdominal muscular contraction and release of oxytocin which in turn accentuates myometrial contraction. The combined forces of intraabdominal and intrauterine pressure propels the fetus through the birth canal. The presence of detached placenta within birth canal initiates further straining and expulsion of the placenta.

44. What is involution of uterus?

Ans. It is the restoration of uterus to its normal non pregnant size and function after parturition. It depend on myometrial contraction, elimination of bacterial infection and regeneration of the endometrium. Post partum female makes a post partum adjustment both in uterus and ovary for restoration of her reproductive capacity. Lochia the uterine discharge that normally occur during post partum period is composed of blood, mucus, fetal membrane, maternal tissue and fetal fluids. The expulsion of lochia and reduction of uterine size are caused by uterine contraction. This is due to sustained release of prostaglandin after parturition which increases uterine and thus promotes involution. By day 50 of post partum about 95% of dairy cows resume ovarian cycle and 40% of beef cows resume ovarian cycle.

Choose the Best Answer

1. Which hormone is used to make immature sperm mature

a) Estrogen b) LH
c) FSH d) Progesterone

2. **Which is engorged with blood in an erection**

a) Corpora cavernosa b) Fiberous envelope
c) Septum pectiniforme d) Integument

3. **Difference between male and female sperm is**

a) Female sperm have a larger head
b) Male sperm are lighter
c) Female sperm are faster
d) Male sperm are weaker
e) a and b

4. **Entire process of sperm formation in bovine is about**

a) 5-6 weeks b) 7-8 weeks
c) 3-4 weeks d) 9-10 weeks

5. **Hyper activation of sperm occurs when**

a) Sperm are introduced into the urethra
b) Sperm are ejaculated into the vaginal canal
c) Sperm begin to interact with the fertilizing layer of an egg cell
d) Sperm reach the cervix

6. **Sperm takes how many weeks to travel through the epididymis**

a) 6-8 b) 1-3
c) 2-4 d) 4-6

7. **Which is not a part of male reproductive organ**

a) Scrotum sac b) Testis
c) Ovary d) Accessory gland

8. **Glans penis of male is equal to which part of female as per sexual homology**

a) Clitoral hood b) Clitoris
c) Clitoral glans d) Clitoral crura

9. **Which part of male is equal to the fallopian tubes of female as per sexual homology**

a) Testis b) Appendix testis
c) Vas deferens d) Seminal vesicle

10. Amount of semen in Boar is about

a) 100ml
b) 250ml
c) 400ml
d) 500ml

11. Testosterone is secreted by

a) Sertoli cells
b) Interstitial cells
c) Spermatozoa
d) All of the above

12. Most important hormone in initiating and maintaining lactation is

a) Estrogen
b) FSH
c) Prolactin
d) None of the above

13. Number of spermatozoa produced from one spermatocyte is

a) 1
b) 2
c) 3
d) 4

14. White scar tissue on ovary representing a former site of an ovarian follicle is called

a) Corpus hemorrhagicum
b) Corpus luteum
c) Corpus albicans
d) Corpuscle

15. When fertilized ovum develops into a solid, spherical mass, it is called

a) Zygote
b) Morula
c) Blastocyte
d) Trophoblast

16. Corpus luteum secretes mainly

a) Progesterone
b) HCG
c) Prolactin
d) Testosterone

17. Which part of female is equal to the penis of male

a) Labia majora
b) Clitoral hood
c) Clitoris
d) Labia minora

18. Some of the strongest muscles of body is found in

a) Uterus
b) Clitoris
c) Cervix
d) Labia majora

19. Part that protects the vaginal and urethral opening is

a) Labia majora b) Labia minora
c) Clitoris d) Urethra

20. Release of LH in female causes

a) Menstration
b) Ovulation
c) Increase of endometrial lining
d) Decrease of endometrial lining

21. When ovaries stop producing estrogen, this cause

a) Ovulation b) Implantation
c) Premenstrual syndrome d) Menopause

22. For invitro embryo production the conditions should be

a) 85%CO_2,5%humidity, 38°C temp.
b) 5%CO_2, 85%humidity, 38°C temp.
c) 38%CO_2, 2,5%humidity, 85°C temp.
d) 85%CO_2,10%humidity,38°C temp.

23. Which is not a part of male reproductive organ

a) Scrotum sac b) Testis
c) Ovary d) Accessory gland

24. Volume of semen in Boar per ejaculation is around

a) 100ml b) 250ml
c) 400ml d) 500ml

25. Ovulation takes place with copulation in

a) Tiger & Dog b) Cat & Dog
c) Cat & Tiger d) Horse & Cattle

26. Which species do not contains sigmoid plexus

a) Cattle b) Horse
c) Swine d) Sheep

27. Which is wrong about part of epididymis

a) Caput-head b) Corpus-body
c) Cauda-tail d) Carpus-head

28. Which is not function of epididymis

a) Production of sperm
b) Maturation of sperm
c) Storage of sperm
d) Transport of sperm

29. Highly fertile environment for sperm is

a) Corpus
b) Caput
c) Cauda
d) Epididymis

30. Common passage for urine and sperm is

a) Vagina
b) Urethra
c) Ureter
d) Uterus

31. Secretion of accessory gland of stallion contains

a) Fructose
b) Citric acid
c) Both
d) None

32. Secretion of accessory gland of domestic ruminants contains

a) Fructose
b) Citric acid
c) Both
d) None

33. Which is not accessory gland of male reproductive system

a) Seminal vesicle
b) Prostate
c) Cowpers
d) Bulbourethral

34. Organ of copulation in male is

a) Vagina
b) Penis
c) Uretra
d) Epididymis

35. Seminiferous tubules are not penetrated by

a) Blood vessels
b) Lymph vesicle
c) Both
d) None

36. Which is called as stem cells

a) Spermatosite
b) Spermatozoa
c) Spermatids
d) Spermatogonia

37. Spermatids are formed in process of

a) Spermatogenesis
b) Spermiogenesis
c) Spermatocytogenesis
d) Spermatidogenesis

38. In spermatogenesis number of mitosis required in bull, ram and buck are

a) 3 b) 4
c) 5 d) 7

39. Spermatogenic waves are related to

a) Sperm formation b) Sperm maturation
c) Oogenesis d) Sprmatidogenesis

40. Best environment for sperm in female reproductive tract is

a) Cervix b) Vagina
c) Fallopian tube d) Uterus

41. Number of follicle develops per estrus cycle is not depends upon

a) Heredity b) Environment
c) Hormone d) Vitamins

42. Reproductive cycle is affected by

a) Heredity b) Environment
c) Hormone d) All

43. Spermatogenesis begins in the

a) Epididymis b) Uterine horn
c) Rete testis d) Seminiferous tubule

44. Sertoli cells produce

a) Mucus
b) Androgen-binding protein (ABP)
c) Testosterone
d) FSH and LH

45. Site of oogenesis is

a) Ovary b) Ovum
c) Fallopian tube d) Uterus

46. In first phase of menstrual cycle

a) Oogonia differentiate into primary oocytes

b) About 20 secondary oocytes begin to enlarge
c) Graafian follicle ruptures
d) Dominant follicle gobbles up all other oocytes

47. During ovulation all of the following occur except

a) Rupture of the Graafian follicle
b) Estrogen production is very low
c) FSH and LH production is high
d) Formation of the corpus luteum

48. Optimal fertilization normally occurs in

a) Vagina
b) Uterus
c) Uterine horn
d) Ovary

49. Human chorionic gonadotropin (hCG)

a) Begins to be produced about 4 weeks post-fertilization
b) Is produced by the corpus luteum after ovulation
c) Rescues and maintains the corpus luteum
d) Signals that a new menstrual cycle should begin

50. Placenta is fully developed by which month of gestation

a) 1st
b) 3rd
c) 5th
d) 7th

51. Fluid filled sac that acts as protective cushion and a waste pail for developing embryo is

a) Yolk sac
b) Chorion
c) Placenta
d) Amnion

52. Blood testes barrier is formed by

a) Tunica albugenia
b) Seroli cells
c) Germinal cells
d) Tunica Vsculosa

53. Fructose is the main component of which accessory sex gland

a) Seminal vesicle
b) Prostate gland
c) Cowper's gland
d) All

54. Placenta type in cow is

a) Diffuse
b) Zonary
c) Discoid
d) Cotyledonary

55. Seminal vesicle is absent in

a) Bull b) Horse
c) Dog d) Boar

56. Fusion of male and female gamete is called

a) Promixing b) Syngamy
c) Uniting d) Mixing

57. Sperm mother cells are

a) Sertollicells b) Leydig cells
c) Both d) None

58. Embryologically male reproductive system develops from

a) Para mesonephric duct b) Mesonephric duct
c) Mullerian duct d) None

59. Embryologically female reproductive system develops from

a) Para mesonephric duct b) Mesonephric duct
c) Mullerian duct d) None

60. Condition in which testes fails to descent to scrotum is called

a) Diapedesis b) Suppression
c) Distension d) Cryptorchidism

61. Sigmoid flexure in penis is absent in which animal

a) Bull b) Ram
c) Horse d) Boar

62. Outer most covering of testes is

a) Tunica vaginalis b) Tunica vascularis
c) Tunica albugenia d) None

63. For effective function of testes, the temperature of testes is

a) Higher than body temperature
b) Lower than body temperature
c) Equal to body temperature
d) None

64. Principal storage organ of sperm in male reproductive system is

a) Testes b) Epididymis
c) Vas difference d) Rete testes

65. Muscle that control the effective length of penis in bull and boar

a) Corpus cavernosum b) Erector penis muscle
c) Ischio cavernous d) Retractor penis muscle

66. Sperm concentration per ejaculation in cock is (millions/ml)

a) 800-2000 b) 2000-3000
c) 3000-7000 d) 200-300

67. Ejaculation volume is highest in which species

a) Cock b) Boar
c) Ram d) Bull

68. Process of formation of spermatozoa from spermatid is called

a) Spermiogenesis b) Spermatocytogenesis
c) Spermatogenesis d) Spermiosis

69. After initial mitosis during spermatogenesis how many mitosis occurs in bull

a) 5 b) 4
c) 3 d) 2

70. How many spermatozoas are formed from a single spermatocytes

a) 4 b) 2
c) 1 d) 0

71. Axoneme is present in which part of sperm

a) Sperm head b) Sperm nucleus
c) Middle piece d) Tail

72. Oviducts are suspended by the ligament

a) Mesosalpinx b) Mesoovarium
c) Mesometrium d) Mesovidium

73. Which is both exocrine and endocrine in nature

a) Testes b) Ovary
c) Pancrease d) All

74. Antrum formation within the egg starts from

a) Primary follicle b) Secondary follicle
c) Tertiary follicle d) All

75. Female genital organ that acts as sperm reservoir

a) Vagina b) Cervix
c) Uterus d) Vulva

76. Testosterone is converted to progesterone in presence of

a) LH b) FSH
c) Both d) None

77. Some time menstrual blood does not clot due to presence of

a) Progesterone b) FSH
c) Plasmin d) Estrogen

78. Antrum formation during folliculogenesis depends upon

a) FSH b) Progesterone
c) Estrogen d) All

79. Animal in which progesterone is secreted from placenta not from corpus luteum during pregnancy

a) Cow b) Sow
c) Bitch d) Mare

80. Urethra, prostate and Bulbourethral gland are developed Embryologically from

a) Wolffian duct b) Genital tubercle
c) Urogenital sinus d) Vestibular fold

81. Ovary looks like cluster of grapes in

a) Cattle b) Sheep
c) Mare d) Sow

82. Bicornuate type uterus is in

a) Cattle
b) Sheep
c) Swine
d) Horse

83. Organ in female genital system that play important role in viable sperm selection is

a) Vagina
b) Cervix
c) Valva
d) Uterus

84. Pregnancy is maintained by hormone

a) Estrogen
b) FSH
c) Progesterone
d) Growth hormone

85. Ovulation in cow is at

a) 10-12 hr after end of estrus
b) 10-12 hr after beginning of estrus
c) 10-12 hr before end of estrus
d) Can not be detected

86. Longest phase in estrus cycle is

a) Estrus
b) Metestrus
c) Diestrus
d) Prostrus

87. Which animal is an induced ovulator

a) Bitch
b) Cow
c) Mare
d) Cat

88. Capacitation of sperm occurs in

a) Epididymis
b) Vas deference
c) Cervix
d) Oviduct

89. Element or ions that helps acrososmal reaction

a) Mg+2
b) Na+
c) Ca+2
d) K+

90. Enzyme hyaluronidase from the sperm helps in dissolving

a) Cumulus cells
b) Zona Pellucida
c) Vitelline membrane
d) All

91. Which hormones helps in mammary gland development

a) Progesterone b) Prolactin
c) Estrogen d) All

92. Gestation period (days) of bovine is

a) 310 b) 299
c) 334 d) 280

93. Hormone which is detected in urine during pregnancy is

a) Estrogen b) Oxytocin
c) Chorionic gonadotropin d) FSH

94. At final stage of gestation which hormone is secreted from fetus

a) Growth hormone b) Cortisol
c) Thyroid d) All

95. Implantation of blastocyst occurs in which layer of uterus

a) Myometrium b) Endometrium
c) Enometrium d) None

96. Chemical compound that allows communication between animals of same species is

a) Hormone b) Pheromone
c) Enzyme d) None

97. During estrus cycle the period of early corpus luteum development is

a) Diestrus b) Proestrus
c) Metestrus d) Estrus

98. During partuirition uterine contraction is by which hormones

a) Estrogen b) Oxytocin
c) Cortisol d) All

99. Ovary is suspended by which ligament

a) Mesometrium b) Mesosalpinx
c) Mesoovarium d) Mesometrium

100. Ovulation fossae is present in the ovary of

a) Bitch b) Cow
c) Sow d) Mare

101. Almond shaped ovary is found in which species

a) Cattle b) Sheep
c) Horse d) Both a & b

102. Each ovary may contain around how many number of follicles

a) 50,000-60,000 b) 75,000-100,000
c) 100,000-200,000 d) 300,000-400,000

103. Bipartite type uterus is in

a) Cattle b) Sheep
c) Swine d) Horse

104. Oviduct is also called as

a) Uterus b) Fallopian tube
c) Isthmus d) Infundibulum

Answers

1. c	2. a	3. e	4. d	5. c	6. d	7. c	8. c	9. b	10. b
11. b	12. c	13. d	14. c	15. b	16. a	17. c	18. a	19. b	20. b
21. d	22. b	23. c	24. b	25. c	26. b	27. d	28. a	29. c	30. b
31. b	32. c	33. d	34. b	35. c	36. d	37. a	38. b	49. b	40. a
41. d	42. d	43. d	44. b	45. a	46. b	47. b	48. c	49. c	50. b
51. d	52. b	53. a	54. d	55. c	56. b	57. a	58. b	59. a	60. d
61. c	62. a	63. b	64. b	65. d	66. c	67. b	68. a	69. b	70. b
71. c	72. a	73. d	74. c	75. b	76. b	77. c	78. a	79. d	80. c
81. d	82. c	83. b	84. c	85. b	86. c	87. d	88. d	89. c	90. a
91. d	92. d	93. c	94. b	95. b	96. b	97. c	98. d	99. c	100. d
101. d	102. b	103. a	104. b						

❑❑❑

CHAPTER-6

Respiratory System

The goal of respiration is to provide O_2 to the tissue and to remove CO_2. To achieve these goal, respiration can be divided into four major functional events as i) **Pulmonary ventilation**: It is the inflow and out flow of our between the atmosphere and wag alveoli, ii) **Diffusion of O_2 and CO_2** between alveoli and blood iii) **Transport of O_2 and CO_2** in the blood and body fluid to and from the cell and iv) **Regulation of Ventilation.** The first breath takes place after birth. Fetal lungs are non functional so during intrauterine life the exchange of gases between fetal blood and mother's blood occurs through placenta. Respiration occurs in two stages as inspiration and expiration. During normal breathing inspiration (inhalation) is active process and expiration is passive process. During inspiration air enters the lungs from inspiration and during expiration air leaves the lungs. While passing through the lungs, the atmospheric air (inspired air) delivers O_2 to blood in pulmonary capillaries and in exchange takes away CO_2 from the blood. Generally respiratory tract is divided into two parts as i) **Upper respiratory tract** which include all the structures from nostril to vocal cord ii) **Lower respiratory tract** that include trachea, bronchi and lungs. Upper respiratory tract include all the structures from nostril to vocal cord. They are n**ostrils, nasal cavities, pharynx, epiglottis** and **larynx.** Primary function of respiratory system is gas exchange, with this primary function of respiratory system the respiratory system has number of non-respiratory functions of body such as **olfaction, vocalization, prevention of dust particles, defense mechanism, maintenance of water balance**, **regulation of body temperature, regulation of acid base balance, anti coagulant function, activation of angiotensin I, synthesis of hormonal sub stances etc.** Inspite of elastic property of lungs tissue and the surface tension in alveoli of lungs the collapsing tendency of lungs are prevented by two factors as **intrapleural pressure** and **surfactants.** There are two types of pressures exerted in the thoracic cavity and lungs during process of respiration they are intra pleural pressure or intra thoracic pressure and intra alveolar pressure or intra pulmonary pressure. **Intra pleural pressure or intra thoracic pressure** is the pressure existing in pleural cavity in between visceral and parietal layers of pleura. The pressure existing in the alveoli of lungs is called intra alveolar pressure or intra pulmonary pressure. Pleural pressure is the pressure of fluid in the space between lung pleura and chest wall pleura. Alveolar pressure is the pressure of air inside the lung alveoli. There are different pulmonary volumes as **Tidal volume**: It is the volume of air inspired or expired with each normal breath. It is almost about 500ml. **Inspiratory reserve volume**: It is the maximum extra volume of air that can be inspired above normal tidal volume. It amounts about 3000ml. **Expiratory reserve volume**: It is maximum extra volume of air that can be expired by forceful expiration above normal tidal expiration. It amount about 100ml. **Residual volume:** It is the volume of air remains in the lungs after the most forceful expiration. This volume is of 1200ml.

Short Questions and Answers

1. What is the function of respiration?

Ans. The goal of respiration is to provide O_2 to the tissue and to remove CO_2. To achieve these goal, respiration can be divided into four major functional events as

i) **Pulmonary ventilation**: It is the inflow and out flow of our between the atmosphere and wag alveoli.

ii) **Diffusion of O_2 and CO_2** between alveoli and blood.

iii) **Transport of O_2 and CO_2** in the blood and body fluid to and from the cell.

iv) **Regulation of Ventilation:** The first breath takes place after birth. Fetal lungs are non functional so during intrauterine life the exchange of gases between fetal blood and mother's blood occurs through placenta.

2. What is inspiration and expiration?

Ans. Respiration occurs in two stages as inspiration and expiration. During normal breathing inspiration (inhalation) is active process and expiration is passive process. During inspiration air enters the lungs from inspiration and during expiration air leaves the lungs. While passing through the lungs, the atmospheric air (inspired air) delivers O_2 to blood in pulmonary capillaries and in exchange takes away CO_2 from the blood. Expiration is passive as here muscle does not require to work rather it is stage of muscle relaxation.

3. What is external respiration and internal respiration?

Ans. Exchange of respiratory gases i.e O_2 and CO_2 between alveoli of lungs and blood is called **external respiration** where as the exchange of gases between blood and tissue is called **internal respiration**.

4. Which part of respiratory tract is called upper respiratory tract and which part is called Lower respiratory tract?

Ans. **Upper respiratory tract** include all the structures from nostril to vocal cord and **lower respiratory tract** include trachea, bronchi and lungs

5. What are the functions of respiratory system?

Ans. Primary function of respiratory system is gas exchange, with this primary function the respiratory system has number of non-respiratory functions of body such as olfaction, vocalization, prevention of dust particles, defense mechanism, maintenance of water balance, regulation of body temperature, regulation of acid base balance, anti coagulant function, activation of angiotensin I, synthesis of hormonal substances.

6. What is lung Compliance?

Ans. It is the magnitude of change in lung volume per unit change in intrapulmonary pressure. This compliance can be considered the opposite of stiffness. A low lung compliance means that the lungs need a greater than average change in intra pleural pressure to change the volume of lung. A high lung compliance means the little pressure differences in intra pleural pressures is needed to change the volume of lung.

7. What are the factor affect compliance?

Ans. Factor affecting lung compliance are **factors within lung** and **factors within chest wall**. Factors within lung are elasticity of lung, volume of lung, degree of congestion, alveolar surface tension and paralysis. Factors within chest wall are alveolar surface tension and elastic fiber of lungs.

8. Factors preventing collapsing tendency of lungs

Ans. Inspite of elastic property of lungs tissue and the surface tension in alveoli of lungs the collapsing tendency of lungs are prevented by two factors as **intrapleural pressure** and **surfactants.**

9. What cause recoil tendency of lungs?

Ans. There is constant tendency of lungs to collapse and in doing so they recoil inward from the thoracic wall. This recoil tendency is due to stretching of elastin and collagen fibers by lung inflation and surface tension of fluid lining the alveoli.

10. What is intra pleural pressure and its significance?

Ans. It is the pressure existing in pleural cavity in between visceral and parietal layers of pleura. It is exerted by the suction of the fluid that lines the pleural cavity. It is also called **intra thoracic pressure** since it is exerted in whole thoracic cavity. Normal value of intra pleural pressure during inspiration is -6 mmHg and this value during expiration is -2 mmHg. Intra pleural pressure has two important functions as it prevents collapsing tendency of lungs which is caused by elastic recoiling of lung tissues and also responsible for venous return.

11. What is surfactant and what is its importance in lungs?

Ans. Agent that is responsible for lowering surface tension of fluid is called **surfactant**. The surfactant present in alveoli of lung is called **pulmonary surfactant**. These surfactants are secreted by two cells as i) Type II alveolar epithelial cells of lungs with are called surfactant secreting alveolar cells or **pneumocytes**. There is presence of microvilli ii) Clara cells present on the bronchioles. Surfactant is a lipoprotein complex formed by phospholipids, proteins and ions. Surfactants reduces surface tension in the alveoli of lung and prevent collapsing tendency of lungs. Surfactants are responsible for stabilization of the alveoli which have tendency to collapse. It plays important role in the inflation of lungs during birth. Surfactant also plays is role in host defence within lungs against infection and inflammation.

12. What are different types of breathing?

Ans. **Eupnea**: It is the state of ordinary quiet breathing

Apnea: It is the condition where there is transient cessation of breathing

Dyspnea: It is difficult or laboured breathing

Hyperpnea: It is the condition of breathing in which frequency, depth or both are increased

Hypopnea: It is the breathing in which frequency, depth or both are decreased

Tachypnea: Itr is excessive rapidity of breathing

Bradypnea: It is abnormal slowness of breathing

Polypnea: It is rapid, shallow, panting type respiration

Anoxia: Literary meaning of it is without oxygen

Hypoxemia: It is decrease in oxygen concentration of arterial blood

Hypercapnea: This condition is increased concentration of CO_2 in arterial blood

Hypocapnea: This condition is decreased concentration of CO_2 in arterial blood

Cyanosis: It is bluish or purplish colouration of skin and mucus membrane. The reflects the dehree of deoxygenetaio of hemoglobin. When observed throughout the body it reflects to improper oxygenation blood but when seen locally it is probably caused by blood flow obstruction.

Asphyxia: It is the condition of hypoxia combined with hypercapnea.

Atelectasis: It is the failure of alveoli to open or remain open and usually involves one or more relatively small areas of lung. The usual cause of atelectasis is occlution of bronchus or bronchioles that supply the area.

Pneumonia: It is acute inflammation of lungs that occurs in all species due to variety of lungs.

13. What is Hypoxia?

Ans. **Hypoxia:** It is decrease of oxygen concentration or decrease in partial pressure of oxygen in air, blood or tissue. Hypoxia are normally of four types as

i) **Ambient hypoxia:** It is the condition in which arterial blood is insufficiently saturated with oxygen because of low oxygen concentration in the atmosphere being breathed. This condition occurs naturally in high altitudes.

ii) **Anemic hypoxia:** It is the condition in which there is decrease in oxygen carrying capacity of blood because of shortage of functioning hemoglobin. The partial pressure of oxygen in arterial blood and the percentage of saturation of the hemoglobin are normal but oxygen delivery to tissue are inadequate.

iii) **Stagnant hypoxia:** It is called ischemic hypoxia in which blood flow through the whole body or tissue is diminised. The oxygen content of arterial blood is normal but the tissue fails to receive enough oxygen because of diminised blood flow.

iv) **Hypotoxic hypoxia:** It is the condition in which cells are unable to use oxygen that is supplied. The amount of oxygen in arterial blood is normal but because the cells are unable to use it, the amount is above normal is venous blood.

14. What is the mechanism of pulmonary ventilation or respiration?

Ans. Lungs can be expanded and contracted in two ways i) By downward and upward movement of the diaphragm to lengthen and shorten the chest cavity and ii) By elevation and depression of the ribs to increase and decrease the antero-posterior diameter of the chest cavity. Normal quiet breathing is accomplished entirely by the first method i.e by the movement of diaphragm. During inspiration contraction of the diaphragm pulls the lower surface of the lungs down ward and during expiration the diaphragm relax. The second method for expanding the lungs is to raise the rib cage because in natural resting position the ribs slant downward thus allowing the sternum to fall backward towards the vertebral coloumn. The most important muscles those raise the ribcage are the external intercostals, sternocleido mastoid muscle, anterior serrate, scelani. Muscle that pull the rib cage downward during expiration are mainly abdominal recti and internal inter costal.

15. What are different pulmonary volumes?

Ans. There are different pulmonary volumes as

i) **Tidal volume**: It is the volume of air inspired or expired with each normal breath. It is almost about 500ml.

ii) **Inspiratory reserve volume**: It is the maximum extra volume of air that can be inspired above normal tidal volume. It amounts about 3000ml.

iii) **Expiratory reserve volume**: It is maximum extra volume of air that can be expired by forceful expiration above normal tidal expiration. It amount about 100ml.

iv) **Residual volume:** It is the volume of air remains in the lungs after the most forceful expiration. This volume is of 1200ml.

v) **Inspiratory capacity**: It is equal to the tidal volume plus inspiratory reserve volume

vi) **Functional residual capacity**: It is equal to expiratory reserve volume plus residual volume. It is the volume of air that remains in lungs at the end of each normal expiration.

vii) **Vital capacity**: It is equal to inspiratory reserve volume plus tidal volume plus expiratory reserve volume.

viii) **Total lung capacity**: It is the maximum volume to which lungs can be expanded with greatest possible effort. It is equal to vital capacity plus residual volume.

16. What is minute respiratory volume?

Ans. It is the total amount of air moved into respiratory passage in each minute. This is equal to the tidal volume times the respiratory rate. Example. Normal tidal volume is 500ml and normal respiratory rate is 12 breaths/min. So minute respiratory volume is 500 X 12= 6000ml/min or 6L/min.

17. What is dead space?

Ans. The part of the respiratory tract like nose, pharynx, trachea, bronchi, bronchioles where gaseous exchange does not takes place is called **dead space**. The air present in these dead space is called dead space air. These dead spaces are of two types as **anatomical dead space** and **physiological dead space. Anatomical dead space** are the space of respiratory system from nose to terminal bronchioles. **Physiological dead space** are on the functional point of view. These include the anatomical dead space with two additional volume which are generally considered wasted ventilation. Under normal condition physiological dead space is equal to anatomical dead space.

18. What is cough reflex?

Ans. Bronchi and trachea are so sensitive to light that very slight amount of foreign matters or other cause irritation and initiate **cough reflex**. The larynx and the point where trachea divides in to bronchi called **carnia** is specially sensitive, as well as terminal bronchioles and alveoli are also sensitive to corrosive chemical stimuli such as sulpher dioxide and chlorine gas.

19. What is sneeze reflex?

Ans. This reflex is similar to cough reflex except that it applies to the nasal passage instead lower respiratory passage. Stimulus for sneeze reflex is irritation in nasal passage so that large amount of the air pass rapidly through the nose thus helping to clear the foreign matter from nasal passage.

20. What are the factors affecting rate of gas diffusion in fluid?

Ans. Factors that affect the rate of gas diffusion in a fluid are solubility of the gas in the fluid, cross sectional area of the fluid, distance through which the gas must diffuse, molecular weight of the gas and temperature of the fluid

All the factors can be expressed in a single formulae as

$$D \alpha \frac{\Delta P X A X S}{D X \sqrt{MW}}$$

Where D= Diffusion rate

ΔP= Partial pressure difference between two ends of the diffusion pathway

A= Cross sectional area of the pathway or fluid.

S=Solubility of the gas in the fluid

D=Distance of diffusion through which the gas diffuse

MW=Molecular weight of the gas.

21. What are the factors affecting rate of gas diffusion through respiratory membrane?

Ans. Diffusion of gases through respiratory membrane is affected by the same factors that affect diffusion of gases through fluids. So the same principle and mathematical formulae is applied to the diffusion of gases through respiratory membrane. Thus the factors that determine the passage of gases through the membranes are i) thickness of membrane ii) surface area of membrane iii) diffusion coefficient of the gas in the substance of the membrane iv) partial pressure difference of the gas between two sides of the membrane.

22. How oxygen is diffused from atmosphere to tissue ?

Ans. Diffusion of oxygen from atmosphere to tissue include the steps like

i) **From atmosphere to alveoli:** The partial pressure of oxygen in the atmosphere is 159 mmHg and in alveoli it is 104 mmHg. Because of this pressure gradient of 55mmHG oxygen easily enters alveoli from atmosphere.

ii) **From alveoli to blood:** Partial pressure of oxygen in pulmonary capillary is 40 mmHg and in alveoli it is 104 mmHg. The pressure gradient is 64mmHg. This pressure gradient facilitate the diffusion of oxygen from alveoli to blood.

iii) **From blood to tissue:** Partial pressure of oxygen in arterial blood is 100mmHg where as partial pressure of oxygen in tissue is of around 30 mmHg. Thus a pressure difference of 70mmHg between blood and tissue cause oxygen to easily diffuse into tissue.

23. How carbon dioxide is diffused from tissue to atmosphere?

Ans. Diffusion of carbon dioxide from tissue to atmosphere include the steps like

i) **From tissue to blood:** Due to continuous metabolic activity CO_2 is produced constantly in tissue. So the partial pressure of CO_2 (PCO_2) is high in tissue and is about 50mmHg where as partial pressure of CO_2 in blood (vein) is about 45 mmHg. The pressure gradient of 5mmHg is responsible for diffusion of CO_2 from tissue to blood.

ii) **From blood to alveoli:** Partial pressure of carbon dioxide in alveoli is 40mmHg, where as in vein blood is 45mmHg. The pressure gradient of 5mmHg is responsible for diffusion of CO_2 from blood to alveoli.

iii) **From alveoli to atmosphere:** In atmospheric air the partial pressure of CO_2 is very insignificant and is about 0.23mmHg, where as in alveoli it is about 40mmHg so CO_2 leaves alveoli easily.

24. How oxygen is transported in blood?

Ans. Oxygen transported by blood from lungs to tissue. Oxygen is transport in blood by two forms as

i) About 97% of oxygen is transported in combination with hemoglobin

ii) Remaining 3% is transported in the dissolved state in water of plasma and cell

i) Transport of oxygen in combination with Hemoglobin

Oxygen combines loosely and reversibly with the heme portion of the hemoglobin. One gram of hemoglobin carries 1.34ml of oxygen that is called as carrying capacity of hemoglobin. The fetal hemoglobin has more oxygen carrying capacity than adult because structurally fetal hemoglobin is different from adult hemoglobin. Normally blood with 15gm% hemoglobin carries only 19 ml percentage of oxygen i.e 19 ml of oxygen in 100 ml of blood.

ii) Transport of Oxygen in dissolve state

At normal atrial PO_2 of 100mmHg about 0.3ml of O_2 is dissolved in 100 ml of plasma and transported. The amount of O_2 transported in this state is negligible.

25. What is Oxygen- hemoglobin dissociation curve?

Ans. The relationship between PO_2 and percentage saturation of hemoglobin with oxygen can be explained graphically and the obtained graph is called oxygen- hemoglobin dissociation curve. Normally in arterial blood leaving from lungs hemoglobin is saturated with oxygen upto 97% and PO_2 in arterial blood is 100mmHg (95mmHg). Conversely in venous blood returning from peripheral tissue the PO_2 is about 40mmHg and the saturation of hemoglobin is about 75%. Under normal condition oxygen-hemoglobin dissociation curve is **'S' shaped or sigmoid shaped**. Lower part of the curve indicates dissociation of oxygen from hemoglobin or reduced blood returning from tissue. Upper part of the curve indicates the acceptance of oxygen by hemoglobin depending upon the partial pressure of oxygen. When PO_2 is 25mmHg, the hemoglobin is saturated about 50% of oxygen. At 40mmHg of PO_2 the hemoglobin saturation is 75% and this saturation becomes 97% when PO_2 is 100mmHg. So it can be calculated that the quantity of oxygen bound with hemoglobin in normal arterial blood (where PO_2 is 100mmHg and hemoglobin saturation is 97%) is 19.4ml/100ml of blood. This quantity of oxygen in vein after returning from peripheral tissue become 14.4ml/100ml of blood (PO_2 is 40mmHg and Hb saturation is 75%). Thus under normal condition 5ml of oxygen is transported from lungs to tissue by each 100ml of blood.

26. What are the factors affecting Oxygen- hemoglobin dissociation curve?

Ans. The Oxygen- hemoglobin dissociation curve is shifted to left or right by various factors. Shift to left indicates association or acceptance of oxygen by hemoglobin i.e increase in affinity of hemoglobin for oxygen and shifting of curve to right indicate dissociation or decrease in affinity of hemoglobin for oxygen. Conditions in which Oxygen-hemoglobin dissociation curve shifted to right are i) decrease in PO_2 of oxygen ii) Increase in PO_2 of CO_2 or increase in concentration of CO_2 iii) increase in hydrogen ion concentration or decrease in pH (from 7.4 to 7.2) iv) increase in body temperature v) increase in 2,3 diphosphoglycerate (DPG). Conditions in which Oxygen-hemoglobin dissociation curve shifted to left are i) in fetal blood–because fetal hemoglobin has got more affinity for oxygen than adult hemoglobin ii) increase in alkalinity cause the curve to shift left and iii) decrease in H+ ion concentration.

27. What are Bohr effect and Halden effect?

Ans. An increase in CO_2 in blood cause O_2 to be displaced from hemoglobin is called **Bohr effect**. This is an important factor in increasing O_2 transport. The reverse is also true i.e binding of O_2 with hemoglobin tends to displace CO_2 from blood. This effect is called **Halden effect.** This is an important factor in promoting CO_2 transport. Bohr effect implies the shifting of O_2-Hb dissociation curve to left which occurs in lungs and shifting to right that occurs in tissue.

28. How carbon dioxide (CO_2) is transported in blood?

Ans. Transport of CO_2 by the blood is not nearly as problematical as transport of O_2. Under normal condition an average of 4ml of CO_2 is transported from tissue to lungs in each 100ml of blood. In arterial blood, volume of CO_2 is 48ml percentage with PCO_2 40mmHg. In venous blood volume of CO_2 is 52ml percentage with PCO_2 is 45mmHg. CO_2 is transported in the blood by four ways as i) in dissolved state, ii) as carbonic acid, iii) as bicarbonate and iv) as carbomino compound.

29. What is CO_2 dissociation curve?

Ans. CO_2 is transported in blood as physical solution and in combination with water, plasma protein and hemoglobin. The amount of CO_2 combine with blood depends on PCO_2. The relationship between PCO_2 and the quantity of CO_2 that combines with blood is demonstrated by a graph called CO_2 dissociation curve. Normal dissociation curve shows that the CO_2 content in blood is 48 ml percentage when PCO_2 is 40mmHg and it becomes 52ml percentage when PCO_2 is 48mmHg, CO_2 content becomes 70ml percentage when PCO_2 is about 100 mmHg.

30. What is respiratory exchange ratio?

Ans. It is the ratio of CO_2 out put to O_2 uptake

$$R = \frac{\text{Rate of } CO_2 \text{ out put}}{\text{Rate of } O_2 \text{ uptake}}$$

R= Respiratory exchange ratio

The value of R changes under different metabolic conditions. When person is exclusively on carbohydrate for body metabolism then R rises to 1. Conversely when the person is using exclusively fat for metabolic energy then R falls to 0.7.

31. How respiration is regulated?

Ans. Respiration is regulated by two mechanisms as neural mechanism and chemical mechanism. **Neural mechanism** involves respiratory centers, afferent nerves and efferent nerves. Respiratory centers is composed of several groups of neurons located bilaterally in the medulla oblongata and pons of the brainstem. It is divided in to three major groups of neurons as dorsal respiratory group, ventral respiratory group and pneumotaxic center. With these three major centers another minor center is present in the lower part of pons called Apneustic center which control intensity of respiration. **Dorsal respiratory group** is located on dorsal portion of medulla oblongata and mainly causes inspiration and basic rhythm of breathing. **Ventral respiratory groups** is located in ventro-lateral part i.e on each side of medulla oblongata which mainly cause expiration and inspiration.

Pneomotaxic center is located dorsally in the nucleus parabrachilis of superior portion of the pons, which mainly controls rate and depth of breathing. **Apneustic center** is presented in the lower part of the pons. Importance of this center is not understood but it is presumed that its association is with pneumotaxic center to control intensity of inspiration. In addition to neural control of respiration there are some **chemical factors** in blood that control respiration. Those chemicals are oxygen, carbon dioxide and hydrogen. Change in the concentration of these chemicals affect respiration. Ultimate goal of respiration is to maintain proper concentration of oxygen, carbon dioxide and hydrogen ion in the tissue.

32. What is Hering-Breuer inflation reflex?

Ans. In addition to neural respiratory control mechanism operating within brainstem sensory signals from lungs also help to control respiration. Most important location is in the muscular portion of the wall of bronchi and bronchioles throughout the lungs contain stretch receptor that transmit signals through vagus nerve into dorsal respiratory group of neurons when lungs become over stretched. These signals affect inspiration in the same way as signals from the pneumotaxic center. When lungs become over inflated these stretch receptors activate a feedback response that switches off the inspiratory ramp and stops further inspiration. This is called **Hering-Breuer reflex**. This reflex is also increase the rate of respiration.

33. What is inspiratory ramp signal?

Ans. Nervous signal that is transmitted to the primary inspiratory muscles mainly diaphragm is not instantaneous burst of action potential. Instead in normal respiration it begins weakly and increase steadily in a ramp manner for about two seconds then it ceases abruptly for about three seconds which stops the excitation of diaphragm and allows elastic recoil of the lungs that cause chest wall for expiration. Next the inspiratory signal begins again for another cycle. This repeats again and again with expiration occurring in between. Thus inspiratory signal is a **ramp signal.**

34. What is differences between avian and mammalian respiration?

Ans. Birds have a larynx, but it is not used to make sounds. Instead, an organ termed **syrinx** serves as the **voice box**. Birds have lungs, but they also have air sacs. Depending upon the species, the bird has seven or nine air sacs. The air sacs of birds extend into the humerus the femur (the thigh bone), the vertebrae and even the skull. Birds **do not have a diaphragm**. Because birds have air sacs that reach into the bones and have no diaphragm, respiratory infections can spread to the abdominal cavity and bones. Bird lungs do not expand or contract like the lungs of mammals. In mammalian lungs, the exchange of oxygen and carbon dioxide occurs in microscopic sacs in the lungs, called 'alveoli.' In the avian lung, the gas exchange occurs in the walls of microscopic tubules, called **'air capillaries**. Respiratory system of birds is more efficient than that of mammals, transferring more oxygen with each breath. Birds have a slower respiratory rate than mammals of similar weight. Respiration in birds requires two respiratory cycles (inspiration, expiration, inspiration, expiration) to move the air through the entire respiratory system. In mammals, only one respiratory cycle is necessary. The air sacs permit a **unidirectional** flow of air through the lungs. Unidirectional flow means that air moving through bird lungs is largely fresh air and has a higher oxygen content. In contrast, air flow is **bidirectional** in mammals, moving back and forth into and out of the lungs. As a result, air coming into a mammal's lungs is mixed with old air that has been in the lungs for a while and this mixed air has less oxygen. So in bird lungs, more oxygen is available to diffuse into the blood.

35. What is respiratory cycle?

Ans. **Air flow** through avian lungs and air sacs during respiration by two inspiration and two expiration called **respiratory cycle**. During the first inspiration, the air travels through the nostrils, also called nares of a bird which are located at the junction between the top of the upper beak and the head. The fleshy tissue that surrounds them in some birds is called the **cere**. As in mammals, air moves through the nostrils into the nasal cavity. From there it passes through the larynx and into the trachea. Air moves through the trachea to the syrinx, which is located at the point just before the trachea divides in two. It passes through the syrinx and then the air stream is divided in two as the trachea divides. The air does not go directly to the lung, but instead travels to the caudal (posterior) air sacs. A small amount of air will pass through the caudal air sacs to the lung. During the first expiration, the air is moved from the posterior air sacs through the ventrobronchi and dorsobronchi into the lungs. The bronchi continue to divide into smaller diameter air capillaries. Blood capillaries flow through the air capillaries and this is where the oxygen and carbon dioxide are exchanged. When the bird inspires the second time, the air moves to the cranial air sacs. On the second expiration, the air moves out of the cranial air sacs, through the syrinx into the trachea, through the larynx, and finally through the nasal cavity and out of the nostrils.

Choose the Best Answer

1. **Significant factor to maintain the normal pH of body fluids is the loss of which gas during external respiration**

   a) Oxygen b) Carbon dioxide
   c) Hydrogen d) Nitrogen

2. **Exchange of gases between the lungs and lung capillaries is called**

   a) Internal respiration b) External respiration
   c) Ventilation d) Breathing

3. **An increase in altitude causes a decrease in gas exchange efficiency because**

   a) Less blood circulates through lungs
   b) There is a decrease in oxygen pressure, therefore less of a gradient into lungs during inspiration
   c) Surface area of alveoli decrease
   d) There are fewer red blood cells in blood at high altitudes

4. **Amount of oxygen that diffuses into the blood/minute depends on**

   a) Oxygen pressure gradient

b) Total functional surface area of the alveolar-capillary membrane
c) Alveolar ventilation
d) All of the above

5. Dalton's Law describes

a) Principles of expansion
b) Laws of partial pressures of gases
c) Laws of temperature difference between partial gases
d) Principles of temperature differences under water

6. In an acidic environment, oxygen splits more readily from hemoglobin. This is referred to as

a) Dalton's law
b) Henry's law
c) Charles law
d) Bohr effect

7. What prevents the lungs from overfilling during normal respiratory movements

a) Carotid chemoreceptors
b) Aortic arch baroreceptors
c) Hering-Bruer reflex
d) Depletion of surfactant

8. Which of the following affect hemoglobin binding to oxygen under physiological conditions

a) pH
b) Temperature
c) Oxygen concentration
d) All of the above

9. Total lung capacity is called as

a) Vital capacity
b) Tidal volume
c) Expiratory reserve volume
d) Inspiratory reserve volume

10. Involuntary breathing is caused by

a) Pituitary gland
b) Exocrine gland
c) Cerebral cortex
d) Medulla oblongata

11. Carbon monoxide is dangerous because

a) It binds strongly to hemoglobin, making it unavailable to oxygen
b) It binds strongly to plasma, making it unavailable to carbon dioxide
c) It raises the blood's pH level, causing a person to hyperventilate
d) Carbon monoxide is not harmful

12. Clubbing of the fingers could be a sign of

a) A viral infection
b) An upper respiratory infection
c) Chronic Obstructive Pulmonary Disease
d) Nothing, it's inherited

13. The need to breathe is caused by

a) Decrease in blood pH
b) Increase in blood pH
c) Decrease in blood oxygen levels
d) Decrease in carbon dioxide levels

14. A person more susceptible to Chronic Obstructive Pulmonary Disease may be

a) Long time smoker
b) Long time fireman
c) Child whose parents smoke
d) Farmer that deals with pesticides
e) All of the above

15. Exchange of gases between blood within the capillaries and tissue fluid surrounding the body's cells is called

a) External respiration b) Cell metabolism
c) Cellular respiration d) Internal respiration

16. The medulla oblongata and pons regulate and measure

a) pH level of blood b) Body temperature
c) Amount of O_2 in blood d) Amount of air in lungs

17. Number of alveoli in lung is

a) 300 million b) 300 billion
c) 300 trillion d) 300 thousand

18. In comparision to atmospheric pressure, intrapleural pressure is

a) More pressurized b) Less pressurized
c) Same d) None

19. Hemoglobin gives up oxygen when the environment is more _______

a) Acidic
b) Alkaline
c) Icey
d) Open

20. Sac that surrounds lungs is

a) Diaphragm
b) Visceral Pleura
c) Pulmonary Thorax
d) None of the above

21. Cellular organelle where oxygen is consumed and carbon dioxide is produced

a) Nucleus
b) Cytoplasm
c) Microfilaments
d) Mitochondria

22. Which is a protective reflexes

a) Hiccuping
b) Sobbing
c) Sneezing
d) Itching

23. Gas exchange takes place in

a) Bronchioles
b) Conchae
c) Pulmonary Capillaries
d) Roots of the Lungs

24. Amount of air breath in or out during one respiratory cycle is called

a) Tidal Volume
b) Vital Capacity
c) Expiratory reseerve Volume
d) Residual Volume

25. Acidosis is when blood pH is below

a) 7.05
b) 7.15
c) 7.25
d) 7.35

26. Some air is still left in the lungs even after most forceful expiration is called

a) Tidal Volume
b) Vital Capacity
c) Expiratory reserve Volume
d) Residual Volume

27. An animal with total paralysis of intercostal muscles would still have normal

a) Inspiratory reserve volume
b) Expiratory reserve volume
c) Total lung capacity
d) Vital capacity
e) None of the above

28. Contraction of the abdominal muscles is important in

a) Normal inspiration b) Forced inspiration
c) Normal expiration d) Forced expiration

29. Alveolar surfactant acts to increase pulmonary

a) Surface tension b) Compliance
c) Airway resistance d) Blood flow

30. Administration of which of the following would be expected to cause airway resistance to decrease

a) Muscarinic-cholinergic b) Nicotinic-cholinergic
c) Alpha-adrenergic d) Beta-adrenergic

31. Rate and depth of respiration will increase when

a) Oxygen concentration increase
b) Carbon dioxide concentration increase
c) HCO_3 concentration increase
d) HCO_3 concentration decrease

32. If CO_2 concentration in blood will increase then breathing will

a) Stop b) Decrease
c) Increase d) No change

33. Membrane that surrounds the lungs is called

a) Pericardium b) Pleura
c) Mediastinum d) Mucous membrane

34. Partial pressure of carbon dioxide (PCO_2) is highest in

a) Exhaled gas b) Alveolar gas
c) Systemic arterial blood d) Systemic venous blood

35. Partial pressure of oxygen (P_{O2}) is highest in

a) Exhaled gas
b) Anatomical dead space at the end of expiration
c) Anatomical dead space at the end of inspiration
d) Alveolar gas

36. If an animal breaths through a hose or tube. To keep his tidal volume normal there would have an increased of

a) Dead space
b) Wasted ventilation
c) Systemic arterial carbon dioxide content
d) All of the above

37. At the top of a 3000 meter high mountain, which of the following alveolar partial pressures would be lower than normal

a) Oxygen
b) Carbon dioxide
c) Water vapor
d) Oxygen and Carbon dioxide both

38. Reduction of the pulmonary diffusing capacity to one-fourth of its normal value will affect partial pressures by

a) Decrease PO_2 and decrease PCO_2
b) Decrease PO_2 and increase PCO_2
c) Increase PO_2 and decrease PCO_2
d) Increase PO_2 and increase PCO_2
e) Decrease PO_2 but no change in PCO_2

39 Covering of lung is called

a) Pericardium
b) Peritubule
c) Pleural membrane
d) Peritoneum

40. The resistance to blood flow of the pulmonary vascular bed is lowest

a) When an animal is at rest sitting up
b) When an animal is at rest lying down
c) When an animal is breathing air at high altitude
d) When an animal is exercising maximally

41. **Which of the following may lead to pulmonary edema**
   a) Decrease pulmonary arterial pressure
   b) Decrease in systemic arterial pressure
   c) Decrease volume of blood in the pulmonary circulation
   d) Increase pulmonary capillary permeability to plasma proteins

42. **Higher concentration of what in blood indicates Cyanosis**
   a) Carbon dioxide b) Carbon monoxide
   c) Hydrogenion d) Reduced hemoglobin

43. **Compared with systemic arterial blood, pulmonary arterial blood has a higher**
   a) Oxygen content
   b) pH
   c) Bicarbonate ion concentration
   d) Hb concentration

44. **As blood passes through systemic capillaries, carbonic anhydrase enzyme catalyzes**
   a) Conversion of dissolved CO_2 to carbonic acid
   b) Conversion of carbonic acid to bicarbonate ion
   c) Conversion of gaseous CO_2 to dissolved CO_2
   d) Binding of carbon dioxide to hemoglobin, thus displacing oxygen

45. **Exchange of Oxygen and Carbon dioxide on the respiratory surface occurs through**
   a) Passive transport b) Active transport
   c) Diffusion d) All

46. **Hemoglobin concentration in systemic venous blood of 20 gm/dl blood is**
   a) Above normal b) Below normal
   c) Within the normal range d) All are true

47. **Stroke that destroyed the respiratory center of the medulla lead to**
   a) Immediate cessation of breathing
   b) Apneustic breathing
   c) Ataxic breathing
   d) Rapid breathing

48. The afferent endings for the Hering-Breuer reflex are stretch receptors in the

a) Aorta and carotid arteries
b) Arteries in the cerebral circulation
c) Lungs
d) Heart

49. Stimulation of the reticular activating system of brainstem cause

a) Stimulates ventilation
b) Inhibits ventilation
c) Stimulates inhalation but inhibits exhalation
d) Stimulates exhalation but inhibits inhalation

50. Hyperventilating cause

a) Increases oxygen reserve of systemic arterial blood
b) Decreases pH of systemic arterial blood
c) Decreases PCO_2 of systemic arterial blood
d) Increases brain blood flow

51. Important afferent receptors for respiratory response to systemic arterial carbon dioxide are

a) CO_2 receptors of aortic and carotid bodies
b) H^+ receptors of aortic and carotid bodies
c) CO_2 receptors in medulla of brain
d) H^+ receptors in medulla of brain

52. Which of the following represents a "right-to-left shunt"

a) Pulmonary blood flow through a region of alveolar collapse
b) Blood flow from left ventricle to right ventricle
c) Blood flow from aorta to pulmonary artery through ductus arteriosis
d) All of the above

53. An animal has an alveolar oxygen pressure of 60 mmHg and a systemic arterial oxygen pressure of 56 mmHg. This indicates the condition of

a) Hypoventilation

b) Diffusion limitation
c) Right-to-left shunt
d) Ventilation-to-perfusion nonuniformity

54. Oxygen-Hemoglobin dissociation curve will move to right at

a) Higher CO_2 concentration
b) Higher O_2 concentration
c) Higher HCO_3 concentration
d) Higher Cl- concentration

55. Lack of oxygen equilibration due to diffusion limitation can be evaluated by measuring the

a) Distribution of an inhaled gas mixture containing a radioactive marker
b) Diffusing capacity of CO
c) Diffusing capacity of CO_2
d) Diffusing capacity of N_2 in inhaling air

56. Normal breathing is called

a) Apnoea
b) Eupnoea
c) Dyspnoea
d) Hypoxia

57. Oxygen-Hemoglobin dissociation curve will shift to right on decrease of

a) Acidity
b) CO_2 concentration
c) Temperature
d) pH

58. Amount of air that may still be inspired after inhalation of tidal volume is called

a) Tidal Volume
b) Inspiratory reseerve Volume
c) Expiratory reseerve Volume
d) Residual Volume

59. Amount of air that still be expired after exhalation of tidal volume is called

a) Tidal Volume
b) Inspiratory reseerve Volume
c) Expiratory reseerve Volume
d) Residual Volume

60. Most common substrate of respiration is

a) Fats
b) Amino acids
c) Glucose
d) Sucrose

61. During respiration, the substrate is

a) Reduced
b) Hydrogenated
c) Carbonated
d) Oxidised

62. The percentage of nitrogen in inhaled air and exhaled air are

a) 21 and 21
b) 21 and 78
c) 78 and 21
d) 78 and 78

63. The percentage of carbon dioxide in inhaled air and exhaled air are

a) 0.04 and 4
b) 4 and 0.04
c) 0.04and 0.04
d) 4 and 4

64. The process common to aerobic and anaerobic respiration is

a) Oxidation
b) Glycolysis
c) Kreb's cycle
d) Electron transport chain

65. In higher plants, the gaseous exchange takes place through

a) Stomata
b) Lenticels
c) General surface of some cells
d) All the above

66. In microbes, the gaseous exchange takes place through

a) Stomata
b) Lenticels
c) General surface
d) All the above

67. The energy rich compound generated as final product during respiration is

a) NADH
b) FADH
c) ATP
d) ADP

68. The source of oxygen for the aquatic animals is

a) Atmosphere
b) Water
c) Soil
d) None of the above

69. Glycolysis takes place in

a) Cytoplasm b) Mitochondrial matrix
c) Mitochondrial cristae d) Ooutside the cell

70. Kreb's cycle operates in

a) Cytoplasm b) Mitochondrial matrix
c) Mitochondrial cristae d) Outside the cell

71. Anaerobic respiration takes place in

a) Cytoplasm b) Mitochondria
c) Outside the cell d) Both a and b

72. Instant source of energy is

a) Sucrose b) Glucose
c) Fats d) Amino acids

73. Number of ATP molecules produced during aerobic and anaerobic respiration are

a) 2 and 8 b) 0 and 2
c) 38 and 0 d) 38 and 2

74. Cramps are caused by heavy exercise resulting in the accumulation of

a) Carbon dioxide b) Lactic acid
c) Ethanol d) Heat

75. Anaerobic respiration in the muscles does not produce

a) Lactic acid b) Energy
c) Carbon dioxide d) Both a and b

76. Product of glycolysis is

a) Carbon dioxide and water b) Pyruvic acid
c) Acetyl CoA d) None of the above

77. Lowering of diaphragm results in

a) Inspiration b) Expiration
c) Digestion d) All

78. Energy produced during respiration is stored in

a) Pyruvic acid
b) Carbon dioxide
c) Adenosine monophosphate
d) Adenosine triphosphate

79. Process complementary to respiration is

a) Circulation
b) Photosynthesis
c) Osmoregulation
d) None of the above

80. Respiratory surface should be

a) Permeable
b) Thin
c) Richly supplied with blood vessels
d) All the above

81. Part of the respiratory tract that is responsible for keeping it healthy is

a) Trachea
b) Bronchi
c) Nasal cavity
d) All the above

82. Hiccups can be best described as

a) Forceful sudden expiration
b) Jerky incomplete inspiration
c) Vibration of the soft palate during breathing while sleeping
d) Sign of somebody remembering

83. Snoring can be best described as

a) Forceful sudden expiration
b) Jerky incomplete inspiration
c) Vibration of the soft palate during breathing while sleeping
d) Sound sleep

84. Sneezing can be best described as

a) Forceful sudden expiration
b) Jerky incomplete inspiration
c) Vibration of the soft palate during breathing while sleeping
d) Something you should never do when someone is going out

85. Respiration in addition to producing energy also carry out the function of

a) Producing the major part of body heat
b) Manufacturing food
c) Maintaining water levels
d) All the above

86. Which of the following are the stages of respiration in the correct order

a) Gaseous transport, breathing, tissue respiration and cellular respiration
b) Breathing, gaseous transport, tissue respiration and cellular respiration
c) Breathing, gaseous transport, cellular respiration and tissue respiration
d) Breathing, tissue respiration, cellular respiration and gaseous transport

87. Epiglottis guards the entrance of

a) Pharynx b) Wind pipe
c) Bronchus d) Lungs

88. The expired air differs from the inspired air by

a) It contains more carbon dioxide
b) It contains less oxygen
c) It contains more water vapour
d) All the above

89. Which structure separates thorax from abdomen

a) Lungs b) Heart
c) Diaphragm d) Rib cage

90. Which metallic element is present in hemoglobin

a) Magnesium b) Sodium
c) Iron d) Calcium

91. Muscles responsible for expiration are

a) External inter costal

b) Internal inter costal
c) External inter costal and abdominal
d) Internal inter costal and abdominal

92. Part of the brain that controls respiratory movements is

a) Cerebrum b) Cerebellum
c) Medulla d) Medusa

93. The instrument used to measure the volume of respired gases is

a) Respiroscope b) Spirometer
c) Barometer d) Thermometer

94. Maximum carbon dioxide concentration is in

a) Inspired air b) Expired air
c) Dead space air d) All will be same

95. Complemental air is

a) Inspiratory reserve air b) Expiratory reserve air
c) Tidal volume d) Vital capacity

96. Supplemental air is

a) Inspiratory reserve air b) Expiratory reserve air
c) Tidal volume d) Vital capacity

97. Volume of air that can be taken in and expelled out by maximum inspiration and expiration is

a) Lung capacity b) Vital capacity
c) Tidal volume d) Respiratory volume

98. Which of the following statements is true about lungs

a) Lungs are spongy but not elastic
b) Lungs are spongy and lobed
c) Lungs are lobed but not spongy
d) Lungs do not have any particular shape

99. Final product of anaerobic respiration is

a) Methanol b) Pyruvate
c) Ethanol d) Starch

100. Function of larynx is to

a) Produce sound b) Absorb oxygen
c) Prevent dust d) Sneezing

101. Inflammation of respiratory path cause

a) Bronchitis b) Thrombosis
c) Sneezing d) Emboli

102. Muscles that are responsible for breathing are

a) Voluntary b) Involuntary
c) Cardiac d) Skeletal

103. Total capacity of lungs for accommodation is called

a) Tidal volume b) Complementary
c) Supplementary d) Vital capacity

104. Diaphragm and intercostals muscles contract to help

a) Inspiration b) Expiration
c) Digestion d) Absorption

105. Amount of air that normally goes in and comes out with every breath is called

a) Complementary air b) Vital capacity
c) Tidal volume d) Total air

106. Amount of air that remains within the lungs after a maximum exhalation is called

a) Residual volume b) Expiratory reserve volume
c) Tidal volume d) Vital capacity

107. Membrane that surrounds the lungs is called

a) Pericardium b) Pleura
c) Mediastinum d) Mucous membrane

Answers

1. b	2. b	3. b	4. d	5. b	6. b	7. c	8. d	9. a	10. d
11. a	12. c	13. a	14. e	15. d	16. a	17. a	18. b	19. a	20. b

21. d	22. c	23. c	24. a	25. d	26. d	27. e	28. d	29. b	30. d
31. b	32. c	33. b	34. d	35. c	36. d	37. d	38. e	39. c	40. d
41. d	42. d	43. c	44. a	45. c	46. a	47. a	48. c	49. a	50. c
51. d	52. a	53. a	54. a	55. b	56. b	57. d	58. b	59. c	60. c
61. d	62. d	63. a	64. b	65. d	66. c	67. c	68. b	69. a	70. b
71. a	72. b	73. d	74. b	75. c	76. b	77. a	78. d	79. b	80. d
81. d	82. b	83. c	84. a	85. a	86. b	87. b	88. d	89. c	90. c
91. d	92. c	93. b	94. b	95. a	96. b	97. b	98. b	99. c	100. a
101. a	102. b	103. d	104. a	105. c	106. a	107. b			

❑❑❑

CHAPTER-7

Nervous System

Most important function of the nervous system is to process incoming information in such a way that appropriate motor responses will occur. More than 99% of sensory informations of brain are irrelevant or unimportant. But when the important informations excites the mind, it is immediately channeled into proper integrative and motor region of the brain to cause desired responses. Basic functional unit of nervous system is **neuron**. Central nervous system contains more than 100 billion neurons. Junction point of one neuron to other neuron is called **synapse.** Nervous system have two parts as **sensory part** and **motor part**. A typical neuron has a **cell body** containing a nucleus, one or more branching filaments called **dendrites** which conduct nerve impulses towards the cell body and one long fiber called **axon** that carries impulses away from it. The large fiber are mylinated and small fibers are non mylinated.

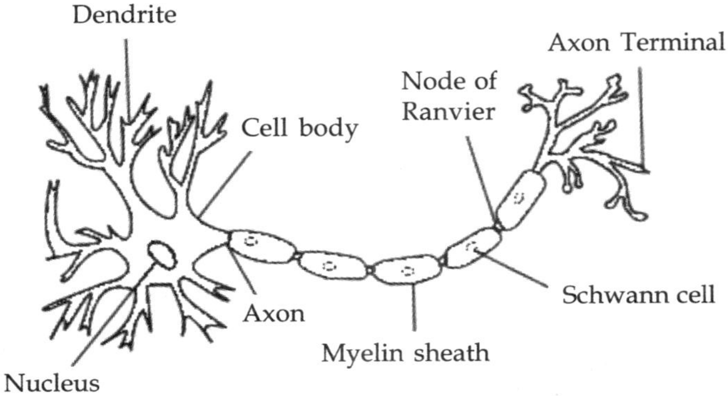

Neuron

The potential difference between outer and inner membrane fiber is **Membrane Potential**. The resting membrane potential of nerve fiber is -90 mv. Nerve signals are transmitted by action potential which are rapid change in the membrane potential that spreads rapidly along the nerve fiber membrane. This membrane potential of a fiber is calculated by a formula as

$$\text{EMF (mV)} = \pm 61 \log \frac{\text{Concentration of ions inside cell}}{\text{Concentration of ions outside cell}}$$

Membrane potential of the fiber is maintained by NA-K pump. Each action potential begins with sudden change from the normal negative membrane potential to a positive potential then ends with equal negative potential. Action potential include three stages as **resting stage, depolarized stage** and **repolarized stage.** Resting stage is resting membrane potential before the action potential begins. During depolarized stage membrane become suddenly permeable to Na^+ ions and allows tremendous Na+ ions flow to interior of axon so the inside negative potential rise rapidly towards positive direction. Within 10000th of a second after the membrane potential highly permeably to Na^+ ions, the Na^+ channels begins to close and the K^+ channels open, then rapidly there is diffusion of K^+ to the exterior part which establish normal negative resting membrane potential called repolarization of membrane. Once the action potential has been elicited at any point on the membrane of a normal fiber, the depolarization process travels over the entire membrane if conditions are right or it might not travel at all if conditions are not right. Nervous system is comprised of two major parts or subdivisions, they are **central nervous system (CNS)** and **peripheral nervous system (PNS).** CNS includes the **brain and spinal cord**. **PNS** consists of the nerves that connect to the brain and spinal cord (cranial and spinal nerves) as well as the **autonomic** (or involuntary) nervous system. Brain consists of three major regions as i) **Fore brain** which includes **cerebral hemispheres** (cerebrum), **hypothalamus** and **pituitary gland** ii) **Hind brain** or **brain stem** that contains **medulla oblongata** and **pons** iii) **Cerebellum** or little brain.

A **reflex** is a rapid automatic response to a stimulus. The path taken by the nerve impulses in a reflex is called a **reflex arc**. Reflex arcs mainly involve three neurons as **sensory neurons, relay neurons** and **motor neurons. Cerebral cortex** is called "higher centres" which concerned with memory, learning, reasoning and intelligence.

Cerebral cortex is the largest portion of the nervous system. The cortex is involved in thought process, memory and analysis of sensory informations. There are several large areas on cortex which are called as **association areas.** Most important association areas are parieto-occipito temporal association area, prefrontal association area and limbic association area.

Nervous system

- Central
  - Spinal cord
  - Brain
- Peripheral
  - Autonomic
    - Sympathetic → Fight/Flight, Speed up/Energizing
    - Para sympathetic → Relaxation, Slow down
  - Somatic

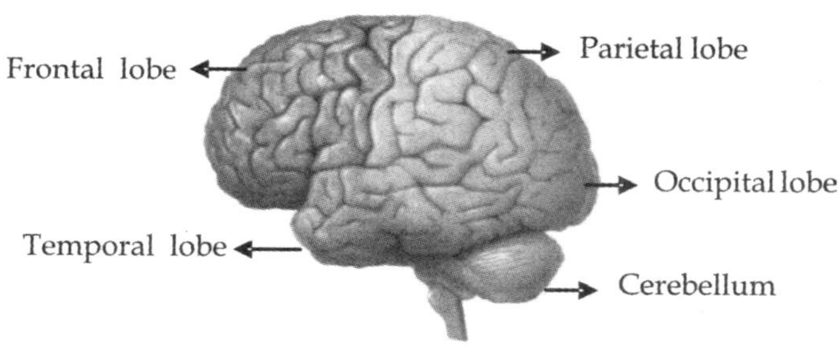

Main sections of brain

Hindbrain or brain stem consists of medulla oblongata, pons and mesencephalon. Brain stem normally control i) respiration ii) cardiovascular system iii) gastro intestinal function iv) many stereotyped movement of the body v) equilibrium vi) eye movement. **Cerebellum** is called **silent area of brain.** This is specially vital to control the rapid muscular activities such as running, playing, typing and even talking. **Peripheral nervous system (PNS)** is a vast network of spinal and cranial nerves that are linked to brain and spinal cord.

The PNS is then subdivided into **autonomic nervous system** and **somatic nervous system**. There are 12 pairs of cranial nerves which arises from brain and brainstem where as spinal nerves are the fibers from CNS to skeletal muscles. The twelve cranial nerves are i) **Olfactory Nerve** for smell ii) **Optic Nerve** for vision iii)**Oculomotor** for looking around iv) **Trochlear** for moving eye v) **Trigeminal** for feeling touch on face vi) **Abducens** to move eye muscles vii) **Facial** to smile, wink, and help us taste viii) **Vestibulocochlear** to help with balance, equilibrium and hearing ix) **Glossopharengeal** for swallowing and gagging x) **Vagus** for swallowing, talking, and parasympathetic actions of digestion xi) **Spinal accessory** for shrugging shoulders xii) **Hypoglossal** for tongue more divided into different regions as muscles. Portion of nervous system that control visceral function of body is called **Autonomic nervous system (ANS)**. The nerves of the autonomic nervous system originate in the spinal cord and pass out between the vertebrae to serve the various organs. This system helps to control arterial pressure, gastro intestinal motility, gastro intestinal secretion, urinary bladder emptying, sweating, body temperature control etc. **Sympathetic system** stimulates the "flight, fright and fight" response that allows an animal to face up to an attacker or make a rapid departure. It increases the heart and respiratory rates as well as the amount of blood flowing to the skeletal muscles. **Parasympathetic system** does the opposite to the sympathetic system. It maintains the normal functions of the relaxed body.

Memory is defined as the act of retaining and recalling past experiences. It is frequently classified as **declarative memory** and **skill memory.** Inspite of frequently classification of memories these memories are also classified commonly as **short term memory, intermediate long term memory** and **long term memory**. **Sleep** is defined as unconsciousness from which the person can be aroused by sensory or other stimuli. It is distinguished from coma which is unconsciousness from which the person can not aroused. Sleep is of two types as **slow wave sleep** and **rapid eye movement sleep**. Most stimulation area causing natural sleep is raphe nuclei in the lower half of pons and medulla. It is known that fibers from raphe nuclei secrete **serotonin** that cause sleep. Other part of medulla and pons called nucleus of tractus solitarus that also promote sleep.

The eyes, ears, nose, tongue and skin are examples of **sense organs**. **Senses** are the physiological methods of perception. All sense organs respond to stimuli by producing nerve impulses that travel to the brain via a sensory nerve. The senses are often divided into two groups as i) **General senses** of touch, pressure, pain and temperature that are distributed fairly evenly through the skin ii) **Special senses** which include the senses of smell, taste, sight, hearing and balance.

Skin is the largest organ of the body not in surface area but in bulk. There are two main components of skin as i) **Epidermis**: It consists of keratinized stratified squamous epithelium and **Dermis**: It is made up of collagenous, elastic and reticular fibers. The structure and thickness of the skin of domestic animals vary according to breed, age and sex. **Sweat gland** is a tubular structure consisting of two parts as i) Deep subdermal coiled portion that secrete sweat ii)A duct portion that passes outward through the dermis and epidermis of the skin Major function of sweat gland is thermoregulation. Another important function of sweat gland is the secretion of pheromones. This is the chemical substance that emit a specific odor when secreted on the surface of the body of an animal which stimulate the olfactory senses of an animal of same species that finally attract both sex of same species during breeding season.

Sebaceous glands in the domestic mammals are associated with the hair follicles and open via pilosebaous canal into upper part of the follicle. They secrete **sebum** a fatty lubricant. At birth the sebaceous glands are large and they become smaller in childhood and grow larger at puberty and adult hood. Sebum provides luster to the hair coat and acts as bacteriostatic and fungistatic agents. Sebum acts as pheromones and olfactant agent.

Eye are organs of **sight**. Eye is composed of eye ball, eyelid, conjunctiva, lacrimal apparatus and extra occular muscle. The **eyeball** contains aqueous humor, iris, lens and vitreous humor. Eye movement is controlled by three pairs of muscles as i) medial and lateral recti that control side to side movement of eye ii) superior and inferior recti that control upward and downward movement of eye and iii)superior and inferior oblique that control rotating of eye ball. Eyes work like a camera. Light rays from an object enter the eye and are focused on the retina at the back of the eye. To stimulate the photo receptors, light must pass through the transparent retinal layers. These photoreceptors are **rods** and **cones**. The retina of domestic mammals contains mostly rods while retina of domestic birds contain mostly cones. The photo sensitive pigments in rods are **rhodopsin** and photo sensitive pigment in cones are called **iodopsin** or **cone pigments** or **colour pigments**. The vision by rods is called **scotoptic vision** and the vision by cones is called **photopic vision**.

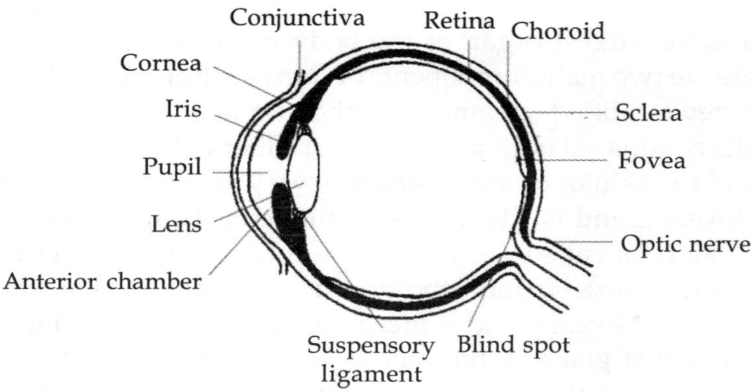

Eye

Ear, the organ of hearing consists of three main regions as **external ear, middle ear** and **inner ear**. External part of ear consists of **pinna** or **auricle** and **external auditory meatus (ear canal)** leading inwards to a thin membrane known as the **ear drum** or **tympanic membrane.** Middle ear consists of a cavity in the skull that is connected to **pharynx** by a long narrow tube called the **Eustachian tube**. Inner ear consists of two main parts as **cochlea (acoustic part)** where sound waves are converted to nerve impulses and **vestibular organ (non acoustic part)** that is associated with the sense of balance and has no role in hearing. Sound waves entering the external auditory meatus or ear canal cause tympanic membrane into vibration. The waves generated are transmitted mechanically accross the tympanic cavity by action of auditory oscicles. The movement of the stapes produce waves in perilymph which cause basilar membrane to vibrate up and down. The range of frequencies that can be detected varies among the species. Human can detects the sounds in the range 20-20 000 Hz (cycles/sec). Loss of hearing or deafness in domestic animals is of two types as i) **sensorineural impairment** and ii) **conduction deafness.** **Audiometer** is the instrument used to determine the nature of hearing disabilities.

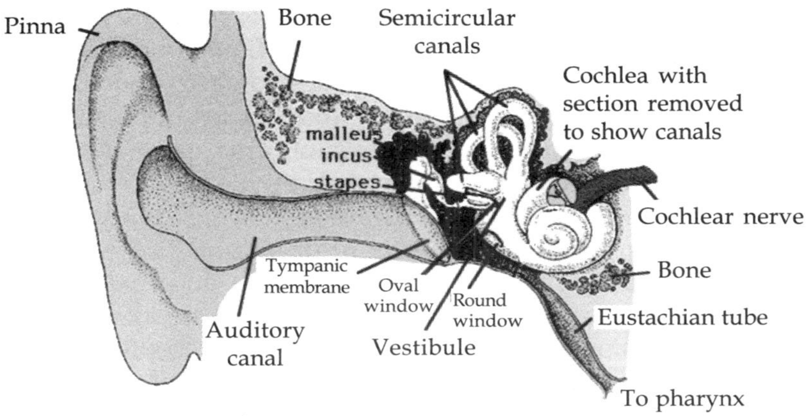

Ear

Short Questions and Answers

1. **What is function of nervous system?**

Ans. **The nervous system has three basic functions as**

i) **Sensory function**: Sensory function is by gathering informations or datas by way of neurons, glia and synapses. This function is to sense stimuli both outside and within the body. These nerves conduct impulses from sensory receptors to the brain and spinal cord.

ii) **Integrative function**: The datas gathered by neurons from sense organs is then processed by way of integration which occurs only in the brain. The impulses from these organs are analyzed and stored as memory. The many different impulses from different sources are sorted, synchronized and co-ordinated and then appropriate response is initiated.

iii) **Motor function**: After the brain has processed the information, impulses are then conducted from the brain and spinal cord to muscles and glands, which is called **motor output**. The motor out put is the response to the stimuli that causes muscles to contract or glands to secrete.

2. **What is Neuron and describe its structure?**

Ans. Basic functional unit of nervous system is **neuron**. Central nervous system contains more than 100 billion neurons. Neurons are cells that have been adapted to carry nerve impulses. A typical neuron has a **cell body** containing a nucleus, one or more branching filaments called **dendrites** which conduct nerve impulses towards the cell body and one long fiber called **axon**, that carries impulses away from it. Many axons have a sheath of fatty material called **myelin** surrounding them. This speeds up the rate at which the nerve impulses travel along the nerve. The cell body of neurons is usually located in the brain or spinal cord while the axon extends the whole distance to the organ that it supplies. A **nerve** is a bundle of axons. A **sensory neuron** is a nerve cell that transmits impulses from a sense receptor such as those in the eye or ear to the brain or spinal cord. A **motor neuron** is a nerve cell that transmits impulses from the brain or spinal cord to a muscle or gland. A **relay neuron** connects sensory and motor neurons and is found in the brain or spinal cord.

3. What is mylinated fiber and why the impulse conduction here is called saltatory conduction?

Ans. The central core of the fiber is called **axon**. The membrane of axon is actually conducts the action potential. Surrounding the axon is a sheath of fatty material called **myelin sheath** about 1-3mm. The fiber containing myelin sheath is called **mylinated fiber**. The large fiber are mylinated and small fibers are non mylinated. The myelin sheath is deposited around axon by schwann cells, i.e the membrane of a schwann cell first envelop the axon, then the cell rotates around the axon many times, lying down multiple layers of cellular membrane containing the lipid substances **sphingomyelin**. This substance is an excellent electrical insulator that decreases ion flow through the membrane about 5000 fold. At the juncture between each two sucessive schwann cells i.e the junction between two myelin sheath the small uninsulated area of 2-3 μm where the ions can flow is called **node of ranvier**. Since no ions can flow through the thick myelin sheath of mylinated fiber they can flow through the node of ranvier. Therefore the action potentials only at nodes and conduct from node to node is called **saltatory conduction.**

4. What is structural classification of neuron?

Ans. This classification of neuron is based on the shape of cell body and relationship of the dendrites to the cell body and axon. By this criteria neurons are classified as

i) **Anaxonic neuron:** These are small and have no anatomical clues to distinguish dendrites from axons. Here all the cell processes look alike. This type of neurons are located in brain and speial organs. Function of this type of neurons are poorely understood.

ii) **Unipolar neuron:** This type of neuron is otherwise called as **pseudounipolar neuron**. Here the dendrites and axon are continuous and basically fused and the cell body lies off to one side. Normally these neurons have one pole and from this pole both axon and dendrite arises. Most sensory neurons of peripheral nervous system are unipolar. Dorsal root ganglion cells are also unipolar.

iii) **Bipolar neuron:** This type of neurons has two distinct processes as one dendritic process and one axon extending from cell body. Bipolar neurons are rare but present in special sence organs where they relay information about sight, smell or hearing. They are smaller than unipolar or multipolar neurons.

iv) **Multipolar neuron:** This type of neuron has a single axon and two or more dendrites. Multipolar neurons are the most common type of neuron in the central nervous system. All the major neurons that control skeletal muscle are multipolar neurons.

5. What is functional classification of neuron?

Ans. The neurons are categorized by function as sensory neurons, motor neurons and interneurons

i) **Sensory neurons:** These neurons are otherwise called as **afferent neurons**. They form the afferent division of the peripheral nervous system and deliver information from sensory receptors to the central nervous system. Sensory neurons are unipolar neurons with processes known as **afferent fibers**, those extend from sensory receptor to the spinal cord or brain. Sensory neurons collect information concerning the external or internal environment through sensory receptors.

ii) **Motor neurons**: These neurons are otherwise called as **efferent neurons**. They form the efferent division of the peripheral nervous system and carry instructions from central nervous system to peripheral tissue. Axons traveling away from central nervous system are called efferent fibers.

iii) **Interneurons:** These neurons are otherwise called as **association neurons**. These neurons are located entirely within the brain and spinal cord. They are responsible for the distribution of sensory information and the coordination of motor activity. Interneurons are also involved with all higher functions such as memory planning and learning.

6. What is synapse?

Ans. It is the junction point from one neuron to other neuron. There are two types of synapses as chemical synapse and electrical synapse.

Chemical synapse: All these synapses are used for signal transmission in the CNS. In these the first neuron secretes a chemical substance at its nerve ending synapse called **neurotransmitter**. This transmitter acts on the receptor of the next neuron to excite, inhibit or modify the sensitivity. More than 50 neurotransmitters have been discovered. Out of these some are acetyl choline (Ach), nor epinephrine (NE), epinephrine, gamma amino butyric acid (GABA), serotonin and glutamine etc.

Electrical synapse: It is formed by gap junction or other similar junctions that action potential are transmitted from one smooth muscle fiber to the next.

7. What are the divisions of nervous system?

Ans. Nervous system is comprised of two major parts or subdivisions, they are **central nervous system (CNS)** and **peripheral nervous system (PNS). CNS** includes the **brain and spinal cord**. **PNS** consists of the nerves that connect to the brain and spinal cord (cranial and spinal nerves) as well as the **autonomic** (or involuntary) nervous system.

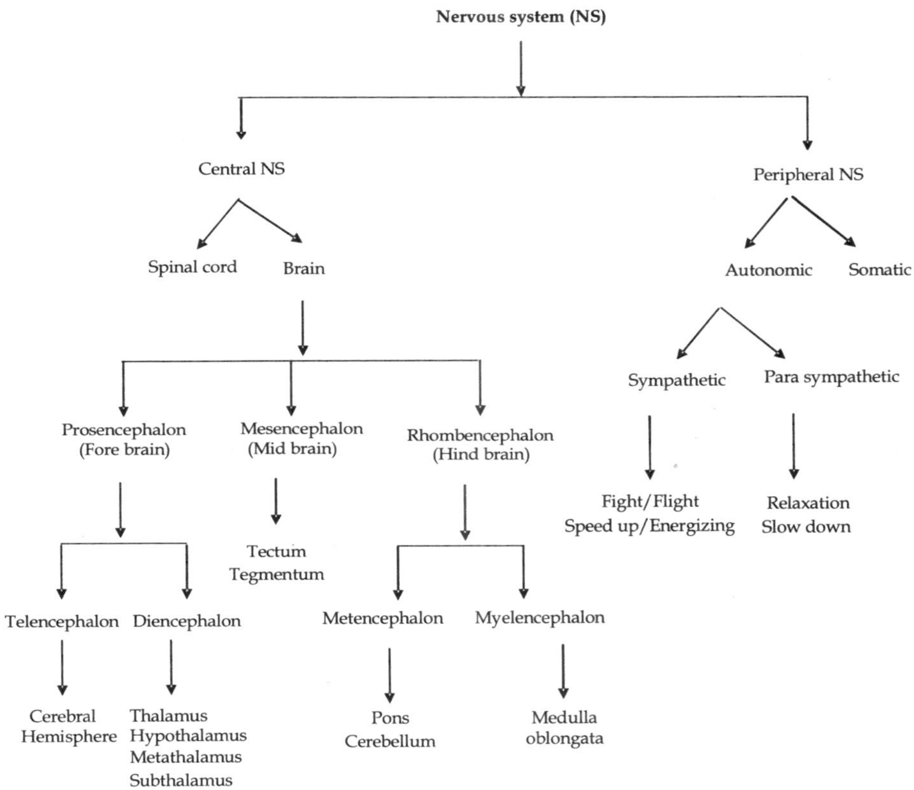

8. What is reflex and reflex arc?

Ans. A **reflex** is a rapid automatic response to a stimulus. When any one accidentally touch a hot object and automatically jerk his hand and goes away, this is a reflex action. Swallowing, sneezing and the constriction of the pupil of the eye in bright light are also all reflex actions. The path taken by the nerve impulses in a reflex is called a **reflex arc**. Reflex arcs mainly involve three neurons. The **stimulus** stimulates the pain receptors of the skin that initiate an impulse in **sensory neurons**. This impulse travels to spinal cord by means of connecting neuron called **relay neurons** situated in the spinal cord. The relay neuron in turn makes a synapse with **motor neurons** that transmit the impulse to the muscles of the affected limb causing them to contract or remove from source of pain. The reflexes has been classified in to number of types as per the muscle shows reflex.

9. What is muscle stretch reflex?

Ans. When a muscle stretch suddenly, excitation of muscle spindle cause reflex contraction of the large skeletal muscle fiber of the same muscle and also of closely allied synergistic muscle. This muscle stretch reflex also called **myotatic reflex**. Muscle stretch reflex can be divided into two components as **dynamic stretch reflex** and **static stretch reflex.** When a muscle is suddenly stretched a strong signal is transmitted to the spinal cord and this causes an instanteneous strong reflex contraction called **dynamic stretch reflex** of the same muscle from which the signal is originated. When this dynamic stretch reflex is over within fraction of second a weaker **static stretch reflex** continues for a prolonged period of time. Importance of static stretch reflex is that it continues to cause muscle contract.

10. What is flexor reflex and withdrawal reflex?

Ans. If any limb is exposed to any stimulating or painful object the flexor muscle of the limb will be contracted and withdrawing the limb from the stimulating object. This type of reflex is called **flexor reflex**. If some part of the body other than limb is painfully stimulated then this part in similar manner will withdraw from the stimulus. Therefore the reflexes of withdrawing different areas of body is called **withdrawal reflex.**

11. What is mark time reflex?

Ans. If an animal is held up from the floor and its legs are allowed to fall downward the stretches on the limbs occasionally elicit stepping reflexes that involves all four limbs. In general stepping occurs diagonally between fore limb and hind limbs. Such walking pattern is called **mark time reflex**.

12. What are the major regions of brain?

Ans. Brain consists of three major regions as

i) **Prosencephalon (Fore brain)** which is further divided into **telencephalon** and **diencephalon. Telencephalon** is consisting of **cerebral hemispheres** (cerebrum) and **diencephalon** is consisting of thalamus, **hypothalamus** and **pituitary gland.**

ii) **Mesencephalon (Mid brain)**

iii) **Rhombencephalon (Hind brain)** which is further divided in to two portions as **metencephalon and myelencephalon.** Metencephalon is formed by **pons and cerebellum** (little brain). Myelencephalon is consisting of **medulla oblongata.** Mid brain, medulla oblongata and pons are together called as **brain stem.**

13. What is the function of Cerebral hemisphere?

Ans. **Cerebral hemispheres** are the masses of brain tissue that sit on the top of the brain. The surface is folded into ridges and furrows called **sulci**. The two hemispheres are separated by a deep groove although they are connected internally by a thick bundle of nerve fibres called **anterior commissure**. The outer layer of each hemisphere is called the **cerebral cortex** where main functions of the cerebral hemispheres are carried out. Cerebral cortex is called **higher centres** which concerned with memory, learning, reasoning and intelligence. Different regions of the cortex are responsible for particular sensory and motor functions, eg. vision, hearing, taste, smell, or moving the fore limbs, hind limbs or tail.

14. What are the important association areas of cerebral cortex and its function

Ans. It is the largest portion of the nervous system. The cortex is involved in thought process, memory and analysis of sensory informations. There are several large areas on cortex which are called as **association areas** because they receive and analyze signals simultaneously from multiple regions of both the sensory and motor areas as well as from sub cortical areas. **Most important association areas** are i) parieto- occipito temporal association area ii) prefrontal association area iii) limbic association area

i) **Parieto- occipito temporal association area** is associated with

a) Analysis of the spatial coordination of body i.e **control. the body movement**

b) **Area of language comprehension** called **wernicke's area**

c) **Visual association area**: This area feeds the visual information conveyed by words read from a book into **wernicke's area**. In absence of this visual association area a person can still have excellent language comprehension through hearing but not through reading.

d) **Area of naming objects**: The name and physical nature of the object are learned through this area by auditory and visual input.

ii) Prefrontal association area

This area is associated with carrying thought process in mind. This area is said to be short term basis "working memory" that are used to analyze each new thought while it is entirely the brain. A special area on the frontal cortex called **broca's area** for word formation. This area is for expressing individual words.

iii) Limbic association area

This area is concerned with behavior, emotion, motivation etc. It is often referred to as the emotional nervous system. It is not only responsible for emotional lives but also for higher mental functions such as learning and memories. There is an area of recognition of faces. Major part of limbic system is **hypothalamus.** Other structures of limbic system are **hippocampus, amygdala, thalamus, cingulate gyrus, fornix** and **parahippocampus**

15. What is major division of hindbrain?

Ans. Hind brain consists of **medulla oblongata, pons** and **cerebellum**. Mesencephalon (mid brain), pons and medulla oblongata are together called as **brain stem. Medulla oblongata** is at the base of the brain and is a continuation of the spinal cord. It carries all signals between spinal cord and brain and contains centres that control vital body functions like basic rhythm of breathing, the rate of the heartbeat and the activities of the gut. The medulla oblongata also coordinates swallowing, vomiting, coughing and sneezing. Brain stem normally control i) respiration ii) cardiovascular system iii) gastro intestinal function iv) many stereotyped movement of the body v) equilibrium vi) eye movement.

16. What is the function of cerebellum (little brain)?

Ans. Apart from cerebral cortex for control of muscle activity, two other brain structures are also essential for normal motor functions, they are cerebellum (little brain) and basal ganglia. **Cerebellum** looks like a smaller version of the cerebral hemispheres attached to the back of the brain. Cerebellum is called **silent area of brain.** This is specially vital to control the rapid muscular activities such as running, playing, typing and even talking. Important function of cerebellum is to sequence the motor activities and also monitor and makes connective adjustments in the body's motor activities. Cerebellum control muscle movement of axial body, neck, shoulder and lips. Anatomically cerebellum has three lobes as i) anterior lobe ii) posterior lobe iii) flocculo nodular lobe. Flocculo nodular lobe is the oldest of all portions of cerebellum and it developed along with vestibular system.

17. What is peripheral nervous system (PNS)?

Ans. PNS is a vast network of spinal and cranial nerves that are linked to brain and spinal cord. It contains sensory receptors which help in processing changes in the internal and external environment. This information is sent to the CNS via afferent sensory nerves. The PNS is then subdivided into **autonomic nervous system** and **somatic nervous system**. The **autonomic nervous system** has involuntary control of internal organs, blood vessels, smooth and cardiac muscles and include sympathetic, parasympathetic and enteric nerves. The **somatic nervous system** has voluntary control of skin, bones, joints, and skeletal muscle and include spinal nerves. **Autonomic nervous system** and **somatic nervous system** function together by way of nerves from the PNS entering and becoming part of the CNS and vice versa. There are 12 pairs of cranial nerves which arises from brain and brainstem where as spinal nerves are the fibers from CNS to skeletal muscles.

18. What are different types of cranial nerves?

Ans. There are twelve pairs of cranial nerves that come from the brain. Each passes through a hole in the cranium (brain case). The twelve cranial nerves are

i) **Olfactory Nerve** for smell

ii) **Optic Nerve** for vision

iii) **Oculomotor** for looking around

iv) **Trochlear** for moving eye

v) **Trigeminal** for feeling touch on face

vi) **Abducens** to move eye muscles

vii) **Facial** to smile, wink, and help us taste

viii) **Vestibulocochlear** to help with balance, equilibrium and hearing

ix) **Glossopharengeal** for swallowing and gagging

x) **Vagus** for swallowing, talking, and parasympathetic actions of digestion

xi) **Spinal accessory** for shrugging shoulders

xii) **Hypoglossal** for tongue more divided into different regions as muscles

19. What are spinal nerves?

Ans. **Spinal nerves** connect the spinal cord to sense organs, muscles and glands in the body. Pairs of spinal nerves leave the spinal cord and emerge between each pair of adjacent vertebrae. The **sciatic nerve** is the largest spinal nerve in the body It leaves the spinal cord as several nerves that join to form a flat band of nervous tissue and gives off branches to the various muscles of this limb.

20. What is autonomic nervous system (ANS) and its major division?

Ans. Portion of nervous system that control visceral function of body is called ANS. **ANS** controls internal body functions that are not under conscious control. The nerves of the autonomic nervous system originate in the spinal cord and pass out between the vertebrae to serve the various organs. This system helps to control arterial pressure, gastro intestinal motility, gastro intestinal secretion, urinary bladder emptying, sweating, body temperature control etc.

21. What are the general organization of the ANS?

Ans. The ANS is activated mainly by centers located in spinal cord, brain stem, cerebral cortex and hypothalamus. The efferent autonomic signals are transmitted to various organs of the body through two major sub divisions called **sympathetic nervous system** and **parasympathetic nervous system. Sympathetic system** stimulates the "flight, fright and fight" response that allows an animal to face up to an attacker or make a rapid departure. Sympathetic nerve fibers originate in the spinal cord between T1 and L2 and pass first in to the sympathetic chain and then to the tissue and organs that are stimulated by sympathetic nerves. Each sympathetic nerve has preganglionic and postganglionic neurons. **Parasympathetic nervous system** does the opposite to the sympathetic system. It maintains the normal functions of the relaxed body. These are sometimes known as the **housekeeping** functions. It promotes effective digestion, stimulates defecation and urination and maintains a regular heartbeat and rate of breathing. These fibers normally leave the CNS through cranial nerves III, VII, IX and X. About 75% of parasympathetic nerve fibers are in vagus nerve. Parasympathetic nerve fiber is also having pre ganglionic and post ganglionic neurons.

22. What is the basic characteristics of sympathetic and parasympathetic functions?

Ans. Sympathetic and parasympathetic nerve fibers secrete one or more neurotransmitter called acetyl cholin and nor epinephrine. Fibers that secrete acetyl choline are called **cholinergic** and the fibers that secrete nor epinephrine are called **adrenergic** (this term is derived from adrenalin which is British name of epinephrine). All pre ganglionic neurons in both sympathetic and parasympathetic system are cholinergic. All post ganglionic neurons of parasympathetic system are also cholinergic. All post ganglionic neurons of sympathetic system are adrenergic. Therefore acetyl choline is called parasympathetic transmitter where as nor epinephrine is called sympathetic transmitter.

23. What is function of sweat glands?

Ans. Major function of sweat gland is **thermoregulation**. After vigorous exercise sweat comes profusely and heat loss from the body surface by evaporation of sweat. But in dog body heat is lost through panting and evaporation. Panting and salivation are the two most important process for controlling body temperature in animals that have limited number of sweat glands. An increase in body temperature in hot weather is a common phenomena in animals while the body temperature of human is kept normal by superbly developed sweating mechanism. Another important function of sweat gland is the secretion of pheromones. This is the chemical substance that emit a specific odor when secreted on the surface of the body of an animal which stimulate the olfactory senses of an animal of same species that finally attract both sex of same species during breeding season. The gland secrete pheromones called **scent glands**.

24. What is sebum and its function?

Ans. Sebum a fatty lubricant secreted from sebaceous glands in the domestic mammals and are associated with the hair follicles which open via pilosebaous canal into upper part of the follicle. The perianal or circum anal glands of dogs are modified sebaceous glands. They are present in both sexes at birth but best developed after puberty forming a ring around anus. Sebaceous gland in dog is similar to that of human being. In cats this gland complexes are dispersed in the connective tissue of the wall of the anal sac at fairly regular intervals. In new born pigs the sebaceous glands are rudimentary but may still contain functional cells. In sheep these glands are associated with the upper third of the wool or hair follicle. In cattle the size of the sebaceous gland is inversely proportional to hair density. They are highly developed in the perianal region and at the horn, hoof and the middle margine but absent in the hairless areas. In goat this gland open independently of the hair follicle in the perianal region and on the eyelid. **Sebum** provides luster to the hair coat andalso acts as bacteriostatic and fungistatic agents. Sebum acts as pheromones and olfactant agent.

25. What is memory and different types of memory?

Ans. Memory is defined as the act of retaining and recalling past experiences. Physiologically it is caused by changes in the sensitivity of synaptic transmission between neurons as result of previous neural activity. Brain areas such as the hippocampus, amygdala, striatum or mammillary bodies are thought to be involved in memory. Memories are frequently classified according to the type of information that is stored. As per this classification memories are of two types as **declarative memory** and **skill memory. Declarative memory** normally means memory of various details of an integrated thoughts such as memory of important experiences that include memory of surrounding, memory of time relationship, memory of experiences, memory of one's deduction that were left in person's mind. **Skill memory** frequently associated with motor activities of the person's body, such as skills developed by practice including automatic memories to sight of the object, calculate the relationship and speed of the object.

Memories can also be classified as **short term memory, intermediate long term memory** and **long term memory**. **Short term memory** is typified by one's memory to seven to ten numbers like as phone number for a few seconds or minutes. Short term memory is due to presynaptic facilitation or inhibition because of release of neurotransmitter that cause facilitation or inhibition. **Intermediate long term memory** can be resulted from temporary chemical or physical changes or both either in presynaptic terminal or postsynaptic terminal. This changes persists for few minutes to several weeks. **Long term memory** is generally believed to result from actual structural changes instead chemical changes at the synapse that cause either enhance or suppress of signal conduction. There is no demarcation between intermediate long term memory and long term memory.

26. What is sleep and types of sleep?

Ans. Sleep is defined as unconsciousness from which the person can be aroused by sensory or other stimuli. It is distinguished from coma which is unconsciousness from which the person can not aroused. Normally sleep is of two types i.e during sleep a person goes through two types of sleep that alternate with each other. They are **slow wave sleep** and **rapid eye movement sleep**.

27. What are characteristics of slow wave sleep and rapid eye movement sleep?

Ans. **In Slow wave sleep** brain waves are large but very slow. It is dreamless sleep. Neurotransmitter serotonin is secreted during slow wave sleep. **Rapid eye movement (REM) sleep** is otherwise called as **paradoxical sleep**. In this type of sleep the eye undergoes rapid movement despite the fact that the person is still asleep. Neurotransmitter nor epinephrine is secreted in rapid eye movement sleep. Most of the sleep is of slow wave sleep which is deep restful sleep where as REM is episodic type and this type is not restful. It is usually associated with dreaming.

Character of REM sleep

i) There is active dreaming and active bodily movement.

ii) Person feels more difficult to arouse by deep slow wave sleep but wake spontaneously during REM sleep.

iii) Heart rate and respiration rate becomes irregular during REM.

iv) There is rapid eye movement in REM sleep.

v) Brain is highly active during REM and all brain metabolism may be increased as much as 20%.

vi) REM sleep is called paradoxical sleep as the person can still be asleep despite marked activity of brain.

28. What is mechanism of sleep?

Ans. Most stimulation area causing natural sleep is raphe nuclei in the lower half of pons and medulla. Nerve fiber from this nuclei spread locally in the brain stem, thalamus, hypothalamus, limbic system and cerebellum. This nerve fibers also extend downward to spinal cord. It is known that these fibers from raphe nuclei secrete **serotonin** that cause sleep. Other part of medulla and pons called nucleus of tractus solitarus which are innervated by vagus and glossopharyngeal nerve that also promote sleep. So lesions in the raphe nuclei leads to high state of wakefulness. Some times lesion of this anterior hypothalamus can cause intensive wakefulness.

29. What is sense?

Ans. **Senses** are the physiological methods of perception. Sense is a faculty by which outside stimuli are perceived. These stimuli are perceived by the presence of sensory receptors present in different part of body. The senses are often divided into two groups as i) **General senses** of touch, pressure, pain and temperature that are distributed fairly evenly through the skin and ii) **Special senses** which include the senses of smell, taste, sight, hearing and balance.

30. What is macrosmatic and macrosmatic animals?

Ans. There are large difference in ability to detect odours among species. The dog is reported to be able to detect odor of lower concentration than are detected by human being. So dogs are labeled as **macrosmatic**, where as animals that can detect odors but are much less sensitive such as some species of birds are called **microsmatic**. Animals which lacks totally an olfactory apparatus can not smell at all are called as **onosmic.**

31. What are different parts of eye?

Ans. The eyes are organs of **sight**. Eye is composed of eye ball, eyelid, conjunctiva, lacrimal apparatus and extra occular muscle. The **eyeball** contains aqueous humor, iris, lens and vitreous humor. Eyeballs are spherical and situated in deep depressions of skull called **orbits**. They are attached to the wall of the orbit by six muscles, which move the eyeball. Upper and lower **eyelids** cover the eyes during sleep and protect them from foreign objects or too much light and spread the tears over their surface. The fibrous external coat of eye ball consists of an anterior part called **cornea** which is transparent and posterior part called **sclera** which is opaque. The middle coat is composed of **choroid, cilliary body** and **iris**. The lens is suspended from a ring of tissues called **cilliary body** in the transparent aqueous humor anteriorly and transparent vitrous humor posteriorly. **Iris** is a diaphragm that divides the aqueous humor into anterior and posterior chamber.

32. How eye sees?

Ans. Eyes work like a camera. Light rays from an object enter the eye and are focused on the retina at the back of the eye. The cornea, lens and fluid within the eye all help to focus the light. They bend the light rays so that light from the object falls on the retina. This bending of light is called **refraction**. The light stimulates the light sensitive cells of the retina and nerve impulses are produced that pass from optic nerve to the brain.

33. What are different types of defective visions?

Ans. Normal vision of eye is called **emmetropia**.

Hyperopia (Far sightness) is either due to short eye ball or due to weak lens system. By using the mechanism of accommodation a far sight person has to use convex lens.

Myopia (Short sightness) is due to mainly long eye ball. To correct this a concave spherical lens is used.

Cataract is the eye abnormality occurs in older people. A cataract is cloudy or opaque area in the lens. In the early stage of cataract formation, the protein in some of the lens fibers become denaturated and later the same proteins coagulate to form opaque areas in place of normal transparent protein fibers. When a cataract has obscured light transmission becomes so greatly that it seriously impairs vision. This condition can be corrected surgically removal of the lens. When this is done the eye losses a large portion of its refractive power which must be replaced by a powerful convex lens in front of the eye.

Color Blindness or color vision deficiency is the inability to perceive differences between some or all colours that other can distinguish. It is most often of genetic nature but may also occur because of eye, nerve or brain damage or due to exposure to certain chemicals. There are many types of color blindness. The most common variety are hereditary photoreceptor disorders, but it is also possible to acquire color blindness through damage to the retina, optic nerve or higher brain areas.

Night Blindness also known as **nyctalopia**, where it is difficult to see in the dark. Night blindness may exist from birth or may be caused by injury or malnutrition (lack of vitamin A). The most common cause of nyctalopia is retinitis pigmentosa, a disorder in which the rod cells in the retina gradually lose their ability to respond to the light. In congenital stationary night blindness the rods do not work from birth, but as the name implies, sufferers do not get worse.

Day Blindness is also known as **hemeralopia** means inability to see clearly in bright light. The daytime vision gets worse and worse. Night time vision remains unchanged due to the use of rods as opposed to cones (during the day), which get affected by hemeralopia and in turn degrade the daytime optical response.

Glaucoma is the disease of eye in which intra occular pressure becomes pathologically high, sometimes rising to 60-70mmHg. Pressure above 20-30mmHg cause loss of vision when maintained for long time. Extremely high pressure can cause blindness within days or even hour. As the pressure increases optic nerve are compressed. This compression is believed to block axonal flow to the cytoplasm.

34. What is retina and its function?

Ans. Retina is light sensitive portion of the eye that contains the cones which are responsible for colour vision and the rods is mainly responsible for vision in dark. There are ten layers of retina and those layers are i) Pigment layer ii) layers of rods and cones iii) outer limiting membrane iv) outer nuclear layer containing cell bodies v) outer plexiform layer vi) inner layer vii) inner plexiform layer viii) ganglionic layer ix) layer of optic nerve fibers x) inner limiting membrane.

35. What is rhodopsin-retinal visual cycle? Or How excitation of rods occurs?

Ans. Rhodopsin which is otherwise called as **visual purple** is a combination of protein **scotopsin** and a carotenoid pigment **retinal**. This retinal is specific i.e 11-cis retinal which only binds with scotopsin to synthesize rhodopsin. When light energy is absorbed by rhodopsin it converted to **bathorhodopsin**. This bathorhodopsin is an unstable compound which is converted to **lumirhodopsin** within nanoseconds. Lumirhodopsin is then converted to **metarhodopsin I** within microseconds and within milliseconds it is converted to **metarhodopsin II**. Finally metarhodopsin II is converted to scotopsin and trans retinal slowly. Metarhodopsin II is called as activated rhodopsin. All trans retinal formed are reconverted to cis retinal directly by enzyme retinal isomerase. Cis retinal (11-cis retinal) which again recombine with scotopsin to form rhodopsin. Conversion of trans retinal to cis retinal may be indirectly by another way. For this conversion trans retinal first converted to trans retinol (form of vitamin A), then trans retinol is converted to cis retinol by isomerase enzyme. Finally cis retinol is converted to cis retinal. Vitamin A is present both in cytoplasm of rods and pigment layer of retina and always available to form new retinal when needed. Therefore vitamin A is absolutely important for vision. In severe deficiency of vitamin A night blindness occurs because due to vitamin A deficiency there is not formation of adequate retinal therefore the amount of rhodopsin that can be formed also becomes severely depressed and the amount of light available at night is too little to permit adequate vision.

36. What is automatic regulation of retinal sensitivity or Light and dark adaptation?

Ans. If a person is in bright light for a long time large portion of the photochemicals in both rods and cones will have been reduced to retinal and opsins. Further much of the retinal of both rods and cones will have also been converted to vitamin A. Because of these two effects the concentration of the photosensitive chemicals remaining in the rods and cones considerably reduced and the sensitivity of the eye to light is correspondingly reduced. This is called **light adaptation**. Conversely if a person remains in dark for a long time the retinal and opsins in the rods and cones are converted back into light sensitive pigments. Furthermore vitamin A is reconverted back into retinal to give still additional light sensitive pigments. This is called **dark adaptation**.

37. What are different parts of ear

Ans. Ear, the organ of hearing consists of three main regions as **external ear, middle ear** and **inner ear**. **External ear** consists of **pinna** or **auricle** and **external auditory meatus (ear canal)** leading inwards to a thin membrane known as the **ear drum** or **tympanic membrane. Middle ear** consists of a cavity in the skull that is connected to **pharynx** by a long narrow tube called the **eustachian tube**. This links the middle ear to the outside air so that the air pressure on both sides of the eardrum can be kept the same. Within the cavity of the middle ear there are three smallest bones in the body known as the **hammer, anvil** and **stirrup** called **auditory ossicles**. **Inner ear** or **lybrinth** is a complicated series of fluid-filled tubes in the bone of skull which is consists of two main parts as **cochlea (acoustic part)** where sound waves are converted to nerve impulses and **vestibular organ (non acoustic part)** that is associated with the sense of balance and has no role in hearing.

38. What is the mechanism of hearing?

Ans. Sound waves entering the external auditory meatus or ear canal cause tympanic membrane into vibration. The waves generated are transmitted mechanically across the tympanic cavity by action of auditory oscicles. The movement of the stapes produce waves in perilymph which cause basilar membrane to vibrate up and down. Because of the movement of basilar membrane the hair cells or stercocillia present on the surface of the basilar membrane becomes activated because of which there is release of neurotransmitter from the base of the hair cells where it synapse with the fibers of the auditory nerve. This neurotransmitter is the stimulus that initiates the nerve impulse to brain.

Choose the Best Answer

1. Transmission of nerve impulses from one neuron to another is by

a) The second cell releases a chemical transmitter
b) The nerve impulse jumps across where the two cells touch
c) Chemical transmitter is released by the first cell
d) Nerve impulses can pass in both directions

2. During action potential

a) K ions rush into the axon b) Na ions move out
c) Both d) Neither

3. Resting membrane potential is due to

a) Insulating effect of schwann cell
b) Large negatively charged proteins on outside
c) Activity of Na-K pump
d) Opening and closing of Na and K channels

4. Interior surface of the membrane of a resting neuron differ from external surface by

a) Negatively charged and contains less sodium
b) Positively charged and contains less sodium
c) Negatively charged and contains more sodium
d) Positively charged and contains more sodium

5. Beta adrenergic receptors are located in

a) Heart muscle
b) Parasympathetic nervous system
c) Postganglionic neurons of the autonomic nervous system
d) Aautonomic ganglia

6. Junction between one neuron and the next neuron is called

a) Synapse b) Dendrite
c) Neuotransmitter d) Ventricle

7. Very sensitive animals such as dogs are labeled as

a) Macrosmatic b) Microsmatic
c) Onosmic d) Both a & b

8. Resting potential is

a) Excess positive ions accumulate inside the plasma membrane
b) Excess negative ions accumulate inside the plasma membrane
c) Excess positive ions accumulate outside the plasma membrane
d) Both b & c

9. Sensory neurons have

a) Short dendrite and long axon
b) Short dendrite and short axon
c) Long dendrite and short axon
d) Long dendrite and long axon

10. What blocks Acetylcholine receptor sites causing muscle relaxation

a) Novocain
b) Curare
c) Nicotine
d) Nerve gases

11. Transmission across a synapse is dependent on the release of

a) Neurotransmitters
b) Synaptic vesicle
c) Neurons
d) Receptor proteins

12. Motor neurons take messages

a) From the muscle fiber to the central nervous system
b) Away from the central nervous system to the central nervous system
c) That are classified
d) Away from the central nervous system to muscle fiber

13. Medulla oblongata helps to regulate which of the following

a) Breathing
b) Heartbeat
c) Vomiting
d) All of the above

14. Main components of the nervous systems are

a) Synapses and Sprinal cord
b) Neurons and the synapses
c) Brain and the neurons
d) Brain and the spinal cord

15. Somatic nervous system is

a) Part of the sympathetic nervous system
b) Part of the parasympathetic nervous system
c) Part of the autonomic nervous system
d) None of the above

16. Effector organs of the autonomic nervous system includes all of the following except

a) Medulla oblongata
b) Heart
c) Smooth muscles
d) Glands

17. Nerves that innervate lymph nodes to be adrenergic suggest that

a) Parasympathetic nervous system may influence lymph node activity
b) Sympathetic nervous system must act to enhance lymph node activity
c) Parasympathetic nervous system has no effect on lymph node activity
d) Sympathetic nervous system may influence lymph node activity

18. Effector pathway of the autonomic nervous system generally contains

a) One neuron b) Two neurons
c) Three neurons d) Five neurons

19. All preganglionic autonomic neurons secrete

a) Epinephrine b) Acetylcholine
c) Nicotine d) Dopamine

20. All postganglionic neurons bear which receptors

a) Alpha adrenergic b) Beta adrenergic
c) Nicotinic d) Muscarinic

21. Parasympathetic nervous system affects all of the organs except

a) Heart b) Pupillary smooth muscles
c) Salivary glands d) Adrenal glands

22. Sclera and cornea constitute which layer of the eye

a) Retinal tunic b) Vascular tunic
c) Fibrous tunic d) Nervous tunic

23. Night blindness is early sign of

a) Cataracts b) Glaucoma
c) Vitamin A deficiency d) Myopia

24. Sympathetic stimulation of the iris causes

a) Astigmatism b) Pupillary constriction
c) Pupillary dilation d) Glaucoma

25. Cone cells are photoreceptors that

a) Respond to low light levels
b) Respond to colored light
c) Are found in the optic disc
d) Are found in the vascular tunic

26. Region where the lens focuses the image onto the retina is the

a) Optic nerve b) Fovea
c) Pupil d) Blind spot

27. Fluid that fills the posterior chamber of the eye is the

a) Lacrimal fluid b) Vitreous humor
c) Aqueous humor d) Jocular humor

28. Major light absorbing pigment in retinal photoreceptors is

a) Rhodopsin b) Melanin
c) Glutamate d) Chlorophyll

29. Photoreceptors release more neurotransmitters in

a) Bright light
b) Darkness
c) When stimulated by bipolar cells
d) None of the above

30. Tenth cranial nerve is

a) Optic b) Vagus
c) Occulomotor d) Auditory

31. Conduction of nerve impulse along a myellienated nerve fibres is

a) Twisted b) Saltatory
c) Continuous d) Reversible

32. Nerve supplied to the posterior part of the tongue is ______

a) Facial b) Glossopharyngeal
c) Vagus d) Trigeminal

33. Area of Language comprehension is

a) Brocas area b) Prefrontal association area
c) Wernickes area d) All

34. Memory house of brain is

a) Pons b) Spinal cord

c) Cerebral Cortex d) Hypothalamus

35. Axon is that part of nerve cell which appears as

a) Short branch b) Long branch

c) Granule d) Central body

36. Nerve messages enter cell through

a) Dendrite b) Axon

c) Cyton d) Synpse

37. Nissel's granule inside the nerve cell are made of

a) DNA b) Protein

c) RNA d) All

38. Axon fiber is insulated by

a) Myelin sheath b) Sarcolemma

c) Protein d) Lipid

39. Neurotransmitter that is found at the synapse or nerve junction is

a) Adrenalin b) Acetyl choline

c) Epinephrine d) GABA

40. Cells which make up the insulation of nerve fiber

a) Schwann cells b) Epithelial cells

c) Flattened cells d) Columnar cells

41. Functional unit of nervous system is

a) Neuron b) Nephron

c) Axon d) All

42. Human brain contains approximately

a) 10 Billion neuron b) 20 Billion neuron

c) 50 Billion neuron d) 100 Billion neuron

43. Neuron come in contact with other neuron at a place is called

a) Axon b) Dendrie
c) Synapse d) Motor

44. In gliosis the cells that enlarge and proliferate are

a) Osteocytes b) Astrocytes
c) Oligocytes d) Dendrocytes

45. How many neurons in nervous system died during development by process c/a Apoptosis/ Programmed cell death

a) 50% b) 60%
c) 70% d) 80%

46. System required to maintain normal resting membrane potential is called

a) Na – K pump system b) Ca-Mg pump system
c) P-Na pump system d) K-Ca pump system

47. At rest the outside membrane of neuron is

a) Positive than outside b) Negative than inside
c) Negative than outside d) Positive than inside

48. All or none law is applicable to

a) Nerve cell b) Muscle cell
c) All excitable d) None

49. Mode of conduction of mylinnated fiber is

a) Continuous conduction b) Saltatory conduction
c) Both d) None

50. Period of recovery of nerve fiber is called

a) Depolarization period b) Refractory period
c) Repolarization period d) None

51. Proprioceptors respond for stimuli originate in

a) Muscle b) Tendon
c) Both d) None

52. Nociceptors are

a) Pain receptors b) Touch receptors
c) Smell receptors d) All

53. Scratch reflex is mostly seen in

a) Human b) Dog & Cat
c) Sheep d) Goat

54. Ascending tract of spinal cord is mainly

a) Sensory type b) Motor type
c) Both d) None

55. Which is not part of CNS

a) Brain b) Cranial nerves
c) Spinal cord d) All

56. Membrane covering brain and spinal cord is

a) Peritoneum b) Durameter
c) Meninx d) All

57. Potential difference between outside and inside of nerve fiber before excitation is called

a) Action Potential b) Resting membrane potential
c) Spike potential d) All

58. Local potential due to flux of Na+ responsible for initiation of action potential is

a) End plate potential b) Spike potential
c) Action potential d) All

59. Signals to reticular activation system by raphe nucleus sleep are

a) Inhibitory b) Excretory
c) Both d) None

60. Body coordination is function of

a) Nervous system b) Endocrine system
c) Both a & b d) Blood vascular system

61. Minimum strength of stimulus that is must to bring the nerve fibers to state of excitation is

a) Minimum stimulus b) Threshold stimulus
c) Perfect stimulus d) Apparent stimulus

62. Indefatibility is property of

a) Nerve cell b) Muscle cell
c) Both a & b d) None

63. Specific protein for transport system of Calcium is called

a) Globulin b) Albumin
c) Myoglobin d) Calmodulin

64. Place where nerve ending joins the muscle fiber is called

a) Neuromuscular junction b) Synapse
c) Synaptic cleft d) None

65. The sharp rise and fall during impulse transmission is called

a) Membrane potential b) Spike potential
c) Action potential d) All

66. Respiratory center is located in

a) Hypothalamus b) Cerebellum
c) Medulla oblongata d) Pons

67. Fluid present in spinal cord is

a) Spinal fluid b) Lymph
c) CSF d) ECF

68. Which wave is recorded in EEG during deep sleep

a) α wave b) β wave
c) γ wave d) δ wave

69. Paradoxical sleep is also called as

a) Rapid eye movement b) Slow wave sleep
c) Both d) None

70. Cranio-sacral nerve is also called as

a) Para sympathetic nerve
b) Sympathetic nerve
c) Autonomic nervous system
d) None

71. Sweat glands are supplied with which nerve

a) Sympathetic b) Parasympathetic
c) Cranial nerve d) All

72. Functionally sweat gland is _________ in nature

a) Sympathetic b) Parasympathetic
c) Cranial nerve d) All

73. Neurotransmitter that is secreted in rapid eye movement sleep

a) Dopamine b) GABA
c) Serotonin d) Nor epinephrine

74. Neurotransmitter that is secreted during slow wave sleep

a) Dopamine b) GABA
c) Serotonin d) Nor epinephrine

75. A center in brain stem which is responsible to regulate sleep is called

a) Brain stem reticular formation
b) Medulla onlongata
c) Pons
d) All

76. Which part helps in secretion of Cerebro spinal fluid

a) Hypothalamus b) Choroid plexus
c) Medulla d) Brain stem

77. Cerebellum is characterized by numerous folds on its surface called

a) Crest b) Wave
c) Folia d) All

78. **Sleep associated with vivid dreaming and found in children is rapid eye movement sleep**

a) Slow wave type
b) Rapid eye movement
c) Partial sleep
d) All

79. **Thermoregulatory center is in**

a) Medulla oblongata
b) Pons
c) Cerebrum
d) Hypothalamus

80. **Hunger and thirst are controlled by Hypothlamus**

a) Medulla oblongata
b) Hypothalamus
c) Pons
d) Cerebrum

81. **Resting membrane potential for nerve fiber is**

a) -50mV
b) -70mV
c) -90mV
d) -100mV

82. **A neuron receives impulse through**

a) Axon
b) Dendrite
c) Myelin sheath
d) Cell body

83. **Otitis media, the inflammatory and infectious process resulting in the accumulation of fluid in**

a) External ear
b) Middle ear
c) Internal ear
d) All

84. **Instrument used to determine the nature of hearing disabilities is**

a) Tonometer
b) Photometer
c) Audiometer
d) All

85. **The sound frequencies that can be detected in the range**

a) 20-20, 000 Hz
b) 100-50, 000 Hz
c) 500-60,000 Hz
d) All

86. **Scala vestibuli and scala media of ear are separated by**

a) Basilar membrane
b) Tympanic membrane
c) Hair cells
d) Reissner's membrane

87. Scala vestibuli and scala tympani contain fluid called

a) Perilymph b) Endolymph
c) Monolymph d) Ectolymph

88. The fluid in scala media is called

a) Perilymph b) Endolymph
c) Monolymph d) Ectolymph

89. Guttural pouch a remarkable diverticulum of eustachian tube found in which species

a) Equine b) Feline
c) Ovine d) Bovine

90. External audtory meatus is separated from tympanic cavity of middle ear by

a) Basilar membrane b) Tympanic membrane
c) Hair cells d) Reissner's membrane

91. Most activity of the nervous system are initiated by

a) Sensory receptors b) Motor receptors
c) Effectors d) Synapse

92. Important function of the nervous system is

a) to process incoming information for appropriate sensory responses
b) to process outgoing information for appropriate sensory responses
c) to process outgoing information for appropriate motor responses
d) to process incoming information for appropriate motor responses

93. Neuron that transmits impulses from sense receptor to brain or spinal cord is

a) Sensory neuron b) Motor neuron
c) Relay neuron d) All

94. Neuron that transmits impulses from brain or spinal cord to muscle is

a) Sensory neuron b) Motor neuron
c) Relay neuron d) All

95. Neuron that connects sensory and motor neurons is

a) Synapse b) Motor unit
c) Relay neuron d) Sensory unit

96. Once the action potential has been elicited, the depolarization process travels over the entire membrane if conditions are right or it might not travel at all if conditions are not right. This is called

a) Law of impulse transfer
b) Polarization principle
c) Ionic exchange principle
d) All or nothing principle

97. The period during which a second action potential can not be elicited even though a strong stimulus is applied is called

a) Safety factor for propagation
b) Absolute refractory period
c) Refractory period
d) Latent period

98. Major part of brain lies protected within a box of skull called

a) Cranium b) Crebo
c) Cerebrum d) None

99. Membranes covering the fragile brain tissue and spinal cord is called

a) White matter b) Gray matter
c) Cranium d) Meninges

100. Crystal-clear fluid that protects and nourishes the brain tissue is called

a) Synovial fluid b) Cerebrospinal fluid
c) Cranial fluid d) All

101. Medulla oblongata and pons are which part of brain

a) Fore brain b) Mid brain
c) Hind brain d) All

102. Which is the large memory store house of body

a) Cerebral cortex b) Medulla oblongata
c) Pons d) Hypothalamus

103. Conduct of action potentials from node to node is called

a) Continuous conduction b) Saltatory conduction
c) Parallel conduction d) None

104. Which part of the brain is considered as higher brain

a) Medulla oblongata b) Hypothalamus
c) Cerebral cortex d) Pons

105. Rapid automatic response to a stimulus is called

a) Action b) Reaction
c) Impulse d) Reflex

106. Path taken by the nerve impulses in a reflex is called

a) Reflex arc b) Nerve cycle
c) Reflex action d) Reaction

107. When a dog is laid on its side it will make incordinated movement that imply

a) Mark time reflex b) Cord righting reflex
c) Galloping reflex d) Scratch reflex

108. Silent area of brain is

a) Medulla oblongate b) Cerebral cortex
c) Cerebellum d) Pons

109. Sympathetic nerve fibers originate in the spinal cord between

a) T1 and L2 b) T1 and L1
c) T2 and L2 d) T2 and L1

110. Normal functions of the relaxed body is maintained by

a) Autonomic nervous system
b) Sympathetic nervous system
c) Parasympathetic nervous system
d) Cranial nerves

111. Fibers that secrete acetyl choline are

a) Adrenergic
b) Cholinergic
c) Both a & b
d) Nicotinic

112. Fibers that secrete nor epinephrine are

a) Adrenergic
b) Cholinergic
c) Muscarinic
d) Nicotinic

113. Which neurotransmitter is secreted during slow wave sleep

a) Substance P
b) GABA
c) Dopamine
d) Serotonin

114. Paradoxical sleep is otherwise called as

a) Rapid eye movement sleep
b) Slow wave sleep
c) Both a & b
d) None

115. Major function of sweat gland is

a) Thermoregulation
b) Heat production
c) Sweating
d) All

116. Major function of sebum is

a) Thermoregulation
b) Heat production
c) Sweating
d) Luster to hair coat

Answers

1. d	2. d	3. b	4. a	5.a	6. a	7. c	8. a	9. c	10. a
1. c	2. d	3. c	4. a	5. a	6. a	7. a	8. d	9. c	10. b
11. a	12. d	13. d	14. d	15. d	16. a	17. d	18. b	19. b	20. c
21. d	22. c	23. c	24. c	25. b	26. b	27. b	28. a	29. b	30. b
31. b	32. b	33. c	34. c	35. b	36. a	37. c	38. a	39. b	40. a
41. b	42. d	43. c	44. b	45. d	46. a	47. d	48. c	49. b	50. b
51. c	52. a	53. b	54. a	55. b	56. c	57. b	58. a	59. c	60. c
61. b	62. a	63. d	64. a	65. b	66. c	67. c	68. d	69. a	70. a
71. a	72. b	73. d	74. c	75. a	76. b	77. c	78. b	79. d	80. b
81. b	82. b	83. b	84. c	85. a	86. d	87. a	88. b	89. a	90. b

91. a	92. d	93. a	94. b	95. c	96. d	97. b	98. a	99. d	100. b
101. c	102. a	103. b	104. c	105. d	106. a	107. b	108. c	109. a	110. c
111. b	112. a	113. d	114. a	115. a	116. d				

□□□

CHAPTER-8

Excretory System

Kidney perform most important functions by filtering the plasma and removing substances from the filtrate at variable rates depending on the need of body. Ultimately kidney remove or clear unwanted substances from the body or filtrate by excreting them in the urine while returning substances that are needed back to the blood. Claudius Galen a Greek physian was first demonstrated that, urine was formed in the kidney and transmitted them to the bladder by the ureters. Modern theory of urine formation was proposed by Arthur Cushny in 1917. Function unit of kidney is called **nephron**. Nephron varies with species but within species the nephron number is constant. Nephron is derived from a Greek word nephron that means kudney. Kidney can not regenerate new nephrons. Therefore with renal injury, disease, normal aging there is gradual decrease in nephron numbers.

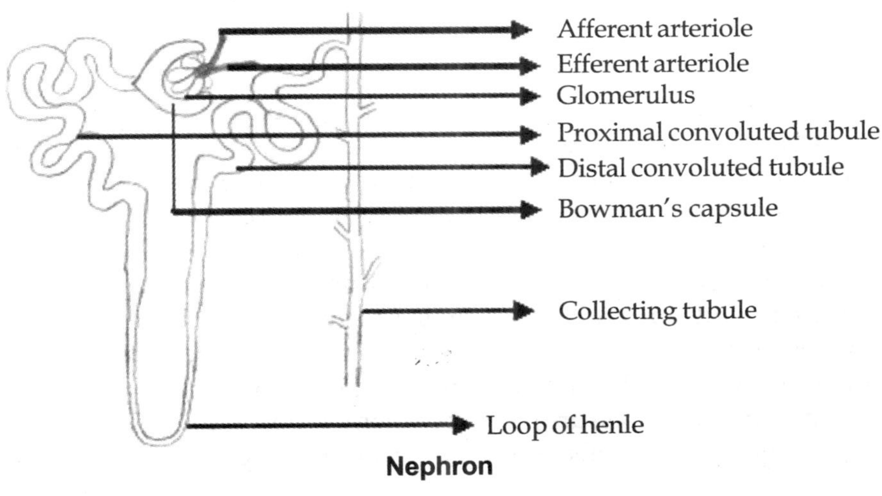

Nephron

Each nephron contains a tuft of glomerular capillaries called **glomerulus** through which large amount of fluid are filtered from the blood. Glomerulus consists of many capillaries connect an **afferent arterioles** with **efferent arterioles**. These glomerular capillaries are covered by epithelial cells and the total glomerulus is encashed in **Bowman's capsule** which is the dilated blind end of nephron. Fluid filtered from glomerular capillaries flows into Bowman's capsule and then goes to **proximal tubule** which lies in the cortex of kidney. From proximal tubule fluid flows in to the **loop of henle** which dips into the renal medulla. Each loop consists of **descending and ascending limbs**. The wall of the descending limb and lower end of ascending limb are very thin and therefore called **thin segment of loop of henle**. After ascending limb of loop of henle has return back to the cortex its wall become thicker and called **thick segment of the ascending limb**. At the end of the thick ascending limb a short segment called **macula densa**, which plays an important role in controlling nephron function. Urine formation include three major steps as i) Glomerular filtration, ii) Tubular reabsorption and iii) Tubular secretion. There are two mechanism required for formation of concentrated urine they are anti diuretic hormone and renal medullary gradient. Kidney has unique anatomical arrangement which are responsible for the development of medullary gradient and for the hyperosmolarity of interstitial fluid in the inner medulla. These arrangements are together called as **counter current system or mechanism**. This counter current mechanism depends on the special arrangement of loop of henle and vasa recta the specialized peritubur capillaries of the renal medulla. In kidney counter current mechanism comprises of two counter current system as counter current multiplier in loop of henle and counter current exchanger in vasa recta.

Regulation of ECF osmolarity and sodium concentration are closely linked because sodium is the most abundant ion in ECF. 90% of the effective osmotic pressure of ECF is due to sodium ion and its associated anions. So sodium plays central role in regulation of ECF osmolarity (Osmoregulation) and volume. In osmoregulation the ratio of sodium to water is being regulated and in volume regulation the absolute amount of sodium and water present are being regulated. Renin-angiotensin-aldosterone system has a role in blood volume homeostasis and maintaining blood pressure. In condition like hypotension (decrease in blood pressure) or hypovolemia (decrease in ECF volume) the juxta glomerular cells of afferent arterioles of glomerulus secrete a proteolytic enzyme **renin** that goes to blood and acts on a plasma protein named **angiotensinogen** (produced in liver) and concert it to **angiotensin I** a 10 amino acid peptide. Within few seconds after formation of angiotensin I it converted to **angiotensin II** a 8 amino acid peptide by converting enzyme secreted from endothelium of lungs. Angiotensin II is an extremely powerful **vasoconstrictor**. Vasoconstriction occurs intensively in arterioles and much less in veins. Constriction of arterioles increases peripheral resistance thereby raising arterial pressure. Mild constriction of the veins promote increase in venous return of blood to the heart thereby helping to increase systemic blood pressure also.

In volume regulation angiotensin II in kidney promotes sodium reabsorption and subsequent water retention. Sodium reabsorption is stimulated directly by angiotensin II in early proximal tubule and indirectly by enhancing **aldosterone** secretion from adrenal cortex. Aldosterone stimulate sodium reabsorption in the cortical and medullary collecting ducts because of which there is increase in ECF volume. **Micturition** is the process by which the urinary bladder empties when it filled. This mechanism involves two main steps as i) bladder fills progressively until the tension on its wall rises above threshold level and ii) first step elicit a nervous reflex called **micturition reflex** that empties the bladder if this fails at least it cause a continuous desire to urinate. The maintenance of relatively constant volume and a stable composition of the body fluid is essential for homeostasis. Homeostasis means the maintenance of static or constant conditions in the internal environment. Total body fluid is mainly distributed between two compartments as intracellular fluid (ICF) and extracellular fluid (ECF). There is another compartment of fluid called transcellular fluid which include synovial fluid, peritoneal fluid, pericardial fluid, cerebrospinal fluid and intra ocular fluid. This transcellular fluid is considered to be a specialized fluid of ECF. Blood is both ECF (fluid in plasma) and ICF (fluid in RBCs). Blood is considered to be a separate fluid because it contained in a chamber of its own i.e the circulatory system.

There are three primary systems in body that regulate the hydrogen ion concentration in the body fluids to prevent acidosis or alkalosis such control systems are

i) The **chemical acid base buffer system of the body** fluids, which immediately combine with acid or base to prevent excessive changes in hydrogen ion concentration.

ii) The **respiratory centre** regulates the removal of CO_2 (and therefore H_2CO_3) from the extracelluar fluid. If the hydrogen ion concentration changes measurably, the respiratory center is immediately stimulated to alter the rate of breathing. As a result, the rate of carbon dioxide removal from the body fluids is automatically changed and this causes the hydrogen ion concentration to return toward normal.

iii) The **kidneys** can excrete either acid or alkaline urine to readjust the extra cellular fluid hydrogen ion concentration. When the hydrogen ion concentration changes from normal during acidosis or alkalosis, the kidneys excrete either acid or alkaline urine, thereby helping to readjust the hydrogen ion concentration of the body fluids back to normal.

Short Questions and Answers

1. What is the function of Kidney?

Ans. There are different functions of kidney like i) Excretion of metabolic waste products and foreign chemicals, ii) Regulation of water and electrolyte balance or homeostasis, iii) Regulation of body fluid osmolality and electrolyte, iv) Regulation of arterial pressure, v) Regulation of acid-base balance, vi) Secretion, metabolism and excretion of hormones, vii) Gluconeogenesis.

2. What are the components of nephron?

Ans. Functional unit of kidney is called **nephron** Each nephron contains a tuft of glomerular capillaries called **glomerulus.** Glomerulus consists of many capillaries connect an **afferent arterioles** with **efferent arterioles**. The glomerulus contains a network of branching and anastomosing glomerular capillaries that compared with other capillaries. These glomerular capillaries are covered by epithelial cells and the total glomerulus is encashed in **Bowman's capsule** which is the dilated **blind end** of nephron. Fluid filtered from glomerular capillaries flows into Bowman's capsule and then goes to **proximal tubule.** From proximal tubule fluid flows in to the **loop of henle** which dips into the renal medulla. Each loop consists of **descending and ascending limbs**. The wall of the descending limb and lower end of ascending limb are very thin and therefore called **thin segment of loop of henle**. After ascending limb of loop of henle has return back to the cortex its wall become thicker and called **thick segment of the ascending limb**. At the end of the thick ascending limb a short segment called **macula densa**, which plays an important role in controlling nephron function. Beyond macula densa fluid enters the **distal tubule** which lies in renal cortex like proximal tubule. This part is followed by connecting tubule and cortical collecting tubule which leads to **cortical collecting duct.**

3. What is the mechanism of urine formation?

Ans. Mechanism of urine formation includes various processes. As when the blood passes to **glomerulus** by afferent arterioles the plasma is filtered into Bowman's capsule and non filterable substances exist through efferent arteriole. The filtrate passes through the tubular portion of nephron. It undergoes various changes like many wanted substances like glucose, amino acids, water, electrolytes are reabsorbed form tubule and the process is called **tubular reabsorption** and unwanted substances are secreted in to the tubule called **tubular secretion or tubular excretion.** When the filtrate passes through the tubular portion of nephron it undergo various changes in quality and quantity. Therefore urine formation include three major steps as i) Glomerular filtration, ii) Tubular reabsorption and iii) Tubular secretion.

4. What is glomerular filtration rate (GFR) and what are the factors affecting glomerular filtration rate?

Ans. The total quantity filtrate formed in all nephrons of both the kidneys in a given time is called **glomerular filtration rate (GFR)**. Factors affecting Glomerular filtration rate are glomerular capillary pressure, colloidal osmotic pressure, hydrostatic pressure in Bowman's capsule,renal blood flow, glomerular capillary filtration coefficient (kf), hydrostatic pressure in glomerulus, constriction or increase in resistance of afferent arterioles, constriction of efferent arterioles, systemic arterial pressure, sympathetic stimulation, permiability of capillary membrane.

5. What are the renal test to assess function of kidney?

Ans. The function of kidney are assessed by various tests which are called renal function test. The renal function tests are of three types as i) Evaluation of renal function by examination of urine, ii) Examination of renal function by examination of blood and iii) Evaluation of renal function by examination of both blood and urine. Urine can be assessed by **composition of urine, specific gravity, colour, odor, consistency and microscopic examination of urine.** Examination of blood to find out the renal function is made by estimation of plasma proteins, urea, uric acid and creatinine.

6. How glomerular filtration rate is measured?

Ans. A substance that is completely or freely filtered at the glomerulus and it should not be neither reabsorbed nor secreted by the tubular epithelium should be used to measure glomerular filtration rate. **Inulin** is a substance that is completely filtered and it is also neither reabsorbed nor is secreted. So inulin is the ideal substance used to measure GFR. **Creatinine** and **radioactive iothalamate** are also used to measure GFR. It is easier than inulin clearance. The normal value of GFR by this method is approximately the same as determined by inulin clearance.

7. How renal plasma flow is measured?

Ans. To measure RPF a substance which is filtered and secreted but not reabsorbed in the tubular lumen should be used. Such substances used to determine RPF is **para amino hippuric acid (PAH).**

8. How renal blood flow is measured?

Ans. To determine renal blood flow value of two factors are necessary they are renal plasma flow and percentage of plasma volume in the blood. Renal plasma flow is measured by using PAH clearance. Percentage of plasma volume is indirectly determined by using PCV. So **renal blood flow= Renal plasma flow/ percentage of plasma in blood.**

9. How concentrated urine is formed?

Ans. There are two mechanism required for formation of concentrated urine they are anti diuretic hormone and renal medullary gradient. **Anti diuretic hormone (ADH)** increases the permeability of distal tubule and collecting ducts to water, thereby allowing these tubular segments to reabsorb water, which finally form concentrated urine. The gradual increase in osmolarity of the renal medullary interstitial fluid is called **medullary gradient.** Kidney has unique anatomical arrangement which are responsible for the development of medullary gradient and for the hyperosmolarity of interstitial fluid in the inner medulla. These arrangements are together called as **counter current system or mechanism**. This counter current mechanism depends on the special arrangement of loop of henle and vasa recta the specialized peritubur capillaries of the renal medulla.

10. What is counter current mechanism?

Ans. Counter current mechanism is the mechanism required for formation of concentrated urine. Counter current mechanism of tubules or vessels exists where the inflow of fluid runs parallel to counter or opposite to and in close proximity to the out flow for some distance. This characteristic is common to the anatomical arrangement of loop of henle and vasa recta. In kidney counter current mechanism comprises of two counter current system as **counter current multiplier in loop of henle** and **counter current exchanger in vasa recta.**

11. What is Barffer's syndrome?

Ans. It is the condition due to defect in transport in the thick ascending limb. It is characterized by chronic sodium loss in the urine with resultant hypovolemia causing stimulation of renin and aldosterone secretion without hypertension, hyperkalemia and alkalosis.

12. What is Renin-angiotensin-aldosterone system?

Ans. Renin-angiotensin-aldosterone system has a role in blood volume homeostasis and maintaining blood pressure. In condition like hypotension (decrease in blood pressure) or hypovolemia (decrease in ECF volume) the juxta glomerular cells of afferent arterioles of glomerulus secrete a proteolytic enzyme **renin** that goes to blood and acts on a plasma protein named **angiotensinogen** (produced in liver) and concert it to **angiotensin I** a 10 amino acid peptide. Within few seconds after formation of angiotensin I it converted to **angiotensin II** a 8 amino acid peptide by converting enzyme secreted from endothelium of lungs. Angiotensin II is an extremely powerful **vasoconstrictor**. Vasoconstriction occurs intensively in arterioles and much less in veins. Constriction of arterioles increases peripheral resistance thereby raising arterial pressure. Mild constriction of the veins promote increase in venous return of blood to the heart thereby helping to increase systemic blood pressure also. In volume regulation angiotensin II in kidney promotes sodium reabsorption and subsequent water retention. Sodium reabsorption is stimulated directly by angiotensin II in early proximal tubule and indirectly by enhancing **aldosterone** secretion from adrenal cortex. Aldosterone stimulate sodium reabsorption in the cortical and medullary collecting ducts because of which there is increase in ECF volume.

13. What is autoregulation mechanism of kidney?

Ans. Renal blood flow (RBF) and GFR are relatively constant regardless of large change in mean atrial pressure. This phenomena is referred to as **autoregulation** of RBF and GFR. It is an intrinsic mechanism and is independent upon out side nerve supply. There are two theories named **Myogenic theory** as well as **Juxta glomerular theory** have been proposed to explain autoregulation.

Myogenic theory: According to this theory increase in blood pressure expand artery and it would responded by contracting. In this way RBF would be decreased and glomerular hydrostatic pressure decreased. This decrease in hydrostatic pressure decreases GFR. A reduction in blood pressure cause less tension and blood vessel would dilate to increase RBF and glomerular hydrostatic pressure with subsequent increased GFR.

Juxta glomerular theory: It is believed that renal hypoperfusion resulting from low blood pressure or blood volume depletion cause JG cells to secrete renin and acts through **Renin-angiotensin-aldosterone system.** The mechanism of tubuloglomerular feed back (TGF) is also associated with the JG theory of autoregulation. TGF refers to the alteration in GFR that can be induced by changes in tubular flow rate. It appears to be mediated by the macula densa cells of the JG apparatus. These cells sense change in delivery of sodium and chloride to their region. Therefore GFR increased because of glomerular hydrostatic pressure, the subsequent increase in macula densa flow and sodium and chloride delivery initiates a response that return GFR and macula densa flow toward normal. The return towards normal is brought about by afferent arteriolar constriction and contraction of mesangium.

14. What is micturition?

Ans. It is the process by which the urinary bladder empties when it filled. This mechanism involves two main steps as i) bladder fills progressively until the tension on its wall rises above threshold level and ii) first step elicit a nervous reflex called **micturition reflex** that empties the bladder if this fails at least it cause a continuous desire to urinate. Smooth muscle of bladder is called **detrusor muscle**. Contraction of deteusor muscle cause emptying of bladder.

15. What is micturition reflex?

Ans. As the bladder fills many superimposed micturition contraction begin to appear. These are result of stretch reflexes initiated by sensory stretch receptors in the bladder wall. Sensory signals from the bladder stretch receptors are conducted to sacral segments of the cord through the pelvic nerves and then reflexes back again to the bladder through parasympathetic nerve fiber by way of the same nerve. This micturition reflex is self generative. Initial contraction of bladder activate stretch receptors to cause still further increase in sensory impulse which cause further increase in reflex contraction of the bladder. Once micturition reflex has occurred but has not succeeded in emptying bladder the reflex usually remain in an inhibited state for few minutes to hour. As the bladder becomes more and more filled micturition reflex occur more and more often and more and more powerful.

16. What is homeostasis?

Ans. **Homeostasis** means the maintenance of static or constant conditions in the internal environment. All the organs and tissues of the body perform functions that help to maintain these homeostatic condition. Fluid intake and output are balanced during steady state condition. The relatively constancy of the body fluids is remarkable because there is continuous exchange of fluid and solutes with the external environment as well as different compartments of the body.

17. What are the ways of daily water intake and loss by body?

Ans. Water is added to the body by two major sources i) By food which is about 2100ml/day and ii) synthesized in body by metabolism which is about 200ml/day. There are different means of water loss from body as **insensible water loss:**There is continuous loss of water by evaporation from the respiratory tract and diffusion through the skin which is about 700ml/day. This insensible water loss through the skin occurs by sweating is about 300-400ml/day and through respiratory tract is around 300-400 ml/day. Fluid loss by sweat is around 100ml/day, water loss in feces is about 100ml/day and water loss by kidney is about 1400ml/day.

18. What are the body fluid compartments?

Ans. Total body fluid is approximately 60% of the body weight. This percentage can be changed depending on age, sex and degree of obesity. As the person grows older the percentage of total body fluid gradually decreases. Total body fluid is mainly distributed between two compartments as intracellular fluid (ICF) and extracellular fluid (ECF). There is another compartment of fluid called **transcellular fluid** which include synovial fluid, peritoneal fluid, pericardial fluid, cerebrospinal fluid and intra ocular fluid. All the fluid outside the cell are collectively called as ECF. This fluid accounts 20% of total body weight. The two greatest compartments of ECF are interstitial fluid which makes over 3/4th of ECF and plasma which makes 1/4th of ECF.

19. What is blood?

Ans. Blood is both ECF (fluid in plasma) and ICF (fluid in RBCs). Blood is considered to be a separate fluid because it contained in a chamber of its own i.e the circulatory system. Blood volume is 7% of total body weight. About 60% of blood is plasma and 40% is RBCs but these percentage can vary in people depending on sex, weight and other factors.

20. What is the way to measure fluid volume in different body compartments?

Ans. The volume of a fluid compartment in the body can be measured by placing an **indicator** substance in the compartment allowing it to disperse evenly throughout the compartment's fluid and then analyzing the extend to which the substance become diluted. In this procedure a small amount of dye or other substance in a syringe is injected into chamber and the substance is allowed to disperse throughout the chamber until it become mixed in equal concentration in all areas. Then a sample of fluid containing the disperse substance is removed and the concentration is analyzed photoelectrically or chemically. If none of the substance leaks out of the compartment, then total mass of the substance in the compartment will be equal to the mass of substance injected.

21. What are the indicators used to determine the volume of specific fluid compartment?

Ans.

i) **Measurement of total body water:** Radio active water ($3H_2O$/tritium) or heavy water ($2H_2O$/deuterium) can be used to measure total body water. Another substance used to measure total body water is antipyrine.

ii) **Measurement of ECF:** The ECF volume can be measured by using radio active sodium, radio active chloride, radioactive iothalamate, thiosulphate ion and inulin.

iii) **Measurement of ICF:** It can be calculated directly by using the formula as Total body water-ECF volume

iv) **Measurement of plasma volume:**To measure plasma volume a substance must be used that does not readily penetrate capillary membrane but remains in the vascular system after injection. Commonly used substance to measure plasma volume is serum albumin labeled with radio active iodine (I^{125}-albumin) and Evans blue dye (T-1824).

v) **Measurement of interstitial fluid volume:** Interstitial fluid can be measured directly by using formula as ECF volume-plasma volume

vi) **Measurement of blood volume:** It can be measured by formula as Plasma volume/1-hematocrit (PCV).

22. What is edema and different types of edema?

Ans. Edema is the presence of excess fluid in the body tissue. In most instances edema occurs mainly in ECF and some times in ICF. Based on the site of accumulation of fluid edema is of two types as intracellular edema and extracellular edema. There are mainly three conditions which are responsible for intracellular edema. They are i) depression in the metabolism ii) malnutrition and iii) inflammation of the tissue. **Extracellular edema** results when there is accumulation of excess fluid in extra cellular spaces. There are four reasons that cause extra cellular edema. Those are i) heart failure ii) renal disease iii) decreased amount of plasma protein iv) lymphatic obstruction.

23. How the hydrogen ion concentration in the body fluids is regulated?

Ans. There are three primary systems in body that regulate the hydrogen ion concentration in the body fluids to prevent acidosis or alkalosis such control systems are

i) **Chemical acid base buffer system of the body** fluids, which immediately combine with acid or base to prevent excessive changes in hydrogen ion concentration.

ii) **Respiratory centre** regulates the removal of CO_2 (and therefore H_2CO_3) from the extracelluar fluid. If the hydrogen ion concentration changes measurably, the respiratory center is immediately stimulated to alter the rate of breathing. As a result, the rate of carbon dioxide removal from the body fluids is automatically changed and this causes the hydrogen ion concentration to return toward normal.

iii) **Kidneys** can excrete either acid or alkaline urine to readjust the extra cellular fluid hydrogen ion concentration. When the hydrogen ion concentration changes from normal during acidosis or alkalosis, the kidneys excrete either acid or alkaline urine, thereby helping to readjust the hydrogen ion concentration of the body fluids back to normal.

Choose the Best Answer

1. Most reabsorption of substances from glomerular filtrate occurs in

a) Glomerulus
b) Collecting tubule
c) Proximal convoluted tubule
d) Ureter

2. Normally kidneys produce _____ liters of glomerular filtrate per day

a) 250 b) 180
c) 110 d) 7.5

3. ADH is produced in

a) Juxtaglomerular cells b) Anterior pituitary gland
c) Hypothalamus d) Posterior pituitary gland

4. At level of ADH in blood, the collecting ducts are

a) Impermeable to water
b) Permeable to protein molecules
c) Permeable to water
d) Permeable to sodium and chloride ions

5. Urine term can correctly be used at

a) Bowman's capsule b) Collecting duct
c) Nephron d) Loop of Henle

6. **Renal cortex contains**

a) Renal pyramids
b) Papillae
c) Calyces
d) None of the preceding

7. **Appearance of glucose in urine**

a) Occurs normally
b) Due to overproduction of angiotensin II
c) Due to hypoglycemia
d) Occurs when the transport carriers for glucose become saturated

8. **Urinary bladder**

a) Has bundles of skeletal muscle in its wall
b) Is connected to the exterior by the ureter
c) Is innervated by the cranial accessory nerve
a) Is located posterior to the pubic symphysis

9. **In proximal convoluted tubule, chloride ions are reabsorbed because of**

a) Active transport
b) Their involvement in calcium retention
c) Electrical attraction of sodium ions
d) High osmotic gradient

10. **Which of the following promotes sodium retention and potassium loss across wall of distal convoluted tubule**

a) Renin
b) Angiotensin II
c) Aldosterone
d) Angiotensin I

11. **Process of micturition**

a) Involves relaxation of the detrusor muscle
b) Requires contraction of the external urethral muscle
c) Is a reflex involving sacral segments of the spinal cord
d) All of the above

12. **Juxtaglomerular cells secrete _____ when there is fall in _____ ion concentration**

a) Renin/Chloride
b) Carbonic anhydrase/Sodium
c) ATPase/Potassium
d) Renin/Sodium

13. Which vessel directs blood into glomerulus

a) Renal artery
b) Afferent arteriole
c) Efferent arteriole
d) Peritubular capillaries

14. Podocytes make up

a) Visceral layer of the nephron
b) Visceral layer of the glomerulus
c) Visceral layer of the renal capsule
d) Visceral layer of the Bowman's capsule

15. Glucose is

a) Filtered, reabsorbed and secreted
b) Filtered and reabsorbed, but not secreted
c) Filtered and secreted, but not reabsorbed
d) Filtered and neither secreted nor reabsorbed

16. If hydrostatic pressure exerted by fluid in capsular space is increased then

a) GFR will increase
b) GFR will decrease
c) No change in GFR
d) May decrease or increase

17. Kidneys process about 180L of blood derived fluids per day but the amount that actually leaves body is

a) 50%
b) 100%
c) 10%
d) 1%

18. Which artery sits on the boundary between cortex and medulla of kidney

a) Lobar
b) Interlobar
c) Arcuate
d) Segmental

19. Fluid in the capsular space is similar to plasma except that it does not contain a significant amount of

a) Glucose
b) Sodium
c) H+
d) Albumin

20. Aldosterone causes

a) Decreased K+ in the urine
b) Increased Na+ in the urine
c) Increased urine output
d) Decreased urine output

21. Creatinine is a

a) Chemical that is typically not secreted
b) Substance typically found in greater amounts in renal arteries than in renal veins
c) Building block for complex carbohydrates
d) All are correct

22. During reabsorption Na^+ crosses the walls of proximal tubule into interstitial fluid by means of

a) Phagocytosis
b) Receptor-mediated endocytosis
c) Simple diffusion
d) Active transport

23. Which is not one of the three external coverings of the kidney

a) Renal capsule b) Adipose capsule
c) Renal fascia d) Renal adventitia

24. Micturition center is located in

a) Pons b) Medulla
c) Cerebellum d) Basal Ganglia

25. Which one creates osmotic gradient in kidney's medulla

a) Vasa recta b) Proximal convoluted tubule
c) Distal convoluted tubule d) Loop of Henle

26. Main solute component of urine is

a) Urea b) Glucose
c) Agglutin d) Urobilinogen

27. Which of the following statement is incorrect

a) Aldosterone stimulates the reabsorption of Na+
b) Aldosterone stimulates the secretion of K+
c) Aldosterone affects water reabsorption
d) Aldosterone is made in the hypothalamus and released from the anterior pituitary

28. Majority of reabsorption occurs in

a) Renal capsule
b) Proximal convoluted tubule
c) Collecting duct
d) Ascending limb of the loop of Henle

29. Which is found in renal medulla

a) Renal pacemaker cells
b) Islets of Langerhans
c) DCT
d) Loop of Henle

30. All of the following are normally found in urine except

a) Glucose
b) Sodium ions
c) Uric acid
d) Urea

31. Which one receives filtrate from glomerulus

a) Proximal convoluted tubule
b) Distal convoluted tubule
c) Bowman capsule
d) Loop of Henle

32. Which is incorrect concerning ADH

a) Its production is regulated by plasma osmolarity
b) Its activity is affected by alcohol
c) It acts on the collecting duct and decreases its permeability to water
d) It is stored in the posterior pituitary

33. Which is not a part of nephron

a) Bowman's capsule
b) PCT
c) DCT
d) Medullary papilla

34 Function of kidney is

a) Release of hormones
b) Maintenance of plasma pH
c) Osmoregulation
d) Gluconeogenesis
e) All of the above

35. Which is part of renal corpuscle

a) Glomerulus b) PCT
c) DCT d) Collecting duct

36. Which is not a stage in urine formation

a) Glomerular filtration b) Glomerular secretion
c) Tubular reabsorption d) Tubular secretion

37. Which is not a means of regulating GFR

a) Regulation via skeletal muscle
b) Regulation via smooth muscle
c) Hormonal regulation
d) Neuronal regulation

38. Increased sympathetic stimulation of afferent arterioles results in

a) Increased filtrate volume per unit time
b) Decreased filtrate volume per unit time
c) Increased GFR
d) Decreased ANP release by macula densa cells

39. Renin is produced by

a) Mesangial cells
b) Macula densa
c) Proximal convoluted tubules
d) Juxtaglomerular cells

40. Nephron is

a) Site of urine storage
b) Functional unit of the kidney
c) Site where ADH is produced
d) Also called the Bowman's capsule

41. Which system cause excretion of soluble nitrogenous wastes

a) Gastrointestinal b) Pulmonary
c) Urinary d) Integumentary

42. Pyramids are areas located within _______ of kidney

a) Cortex b) Pelvis
c) Capsule d) Medulla

43. Ureter directly receives urine from _______ of kidney

a) Cortex
b) Pelvis
c) Medulla
d) Pyramid

44. What is main factor that promotes bladder infections in female

a) Length of urethra
b) Presence of bacteria in rectum
c) Hygiene
d) Dietary factors

45. Structure that is last in the sequence of urine flow is

a) Ureter
b) Kidney
c) Bladder
d) Urethra

46. Outermost structure of kidney is

a) Cortex
b) Medulla
c) Capsule
d) Pelvis

47. Main factor that causes urine to enter urinary bladder is

a) Pressure
b) Peristalsis
c) Gravity
d) Osmosis

48. Inulin is best to use to measure renal clearance because

a) Inulin tastes good, so patients are more apt to be cooperative
b) Inulin is neither reabsorbed or actively secreted into the filtrate
c) Inulin colors the filtrate and thus facilitates scanning of the kidney
d) Inulin is readily available and inexpensive, and thus makes measuring renal clearance fairly simple

49. Peristalsis of detrusor muscle of urinary bladder is controlled by

a) Conscious control of the skeletal muscle
b) Sympathetic nervous impulses
c) Parasympathetic nervous impulses
d) Impulses from the cerebral cortex

50. External urethral sphincter in males is located at

a) Within the urogenital diaphragm

b) Within the penile urethra
c) External urethral orifice
d) Within the prostatic urethra

51. Most small proteins are reabsorbed by

a) Active transport b) Osmosis
c) Facilitated diffusion d) Pinocytosis

52. Hormones those regulate sodium reabsorption and water reabsorption in renal tubule are respectively

a) Aldosterone, antidiuretic hormone
b) Cortisol atrial natriuretic peptide
c) Renin, angiotensin II
d) Antidiuretic hormone, epinephrine

53. Most tubular reabsorption occurs in ________ where microvilli and their numerous carrier proteins, increase surface area available for reabsorption

a) Distal convoluted tubule
b) Proximal convoluted tubule
c) Collecting duct
d) Nephron loop

54 Outermost covering of kidney is

a) Cortex b) Medulla
c) Pelvis d) Capsule

55. Kidneys are located in

a) Pelvic cavity b) Peritoneal cavity
c) Abdominal d) Retroperitoneal

56. Entrance into kidney is called

a) Sinus b) Renal column
c) Hilum d) Pyramid

57. Which structure is first to collect urine

a) Pelvis b) Calyx
c) Ureter d) Urethra

58. Each minor calyx receives urine from

a) Renal papillae b) Pelvis
c) Ureter d) Columns

59. Renal pyramids are located within

a) Column b) Cortex
c) Medulla d) Pelvis

60. Striated appearance of pyramids is caused by

a) Parallel blood vessels b) Microtubules
c) Connective tissue d) Nerve fibers

61. Basic functional unit of kidney is

a) Alveolus b) Renal pyramid
c) Renal pelvis d) Nephron

62. Kidney secretes _______ to stimulate bone marrow activity

a) Renin b) Aldosterone
c) Erythropoietin d) Somatomedin

63. Kidney secretes which enzyme/hormone that raises blood pressure

a) Aldosterone b) Renin
c) Angiotensinogen d) Angiotensin II

64. Function of renal system is

a) Maintain blood pH
b) Regulate blood pressure
c) Control blood concentration
d) All of these

65. How much of cardiac output passes through kidneys

a) 10% b) 25%
c) 50% d) 65%

66. Blood vessel that delivers blood to cortex is

a) Interlobular artery b) Arcuate artery
c) Interlobar artery d) Efferent arteriole

67. **Renal corpuscle is comprised of a glomerulus and ______**

a) Proximal convoluted tubule
b) Bowman's capsule
c) Loop of Henle
d) Distal convoluted tubule

68. **Which section of nephron is after ascending limb of loop of Henle**

a) Descending limb of the loop
b) Proximal convoluted tubule
c) Distal convoluted tubule
d) Collecting duct

69. **Last part of a nephron is**

a) Collecting duct
b) Renal papilla
c) Distal convoluted tubule
d) Glomerulus

70. **Area that secretes renin into blood is**

a) Macula densa
b) Juxtaglomerular apparatus
c) Juxtaglomerular cells
d) Cortical nephron

71. **Blood vessel that conveys blood out of the nephron is**

a) Efferent arteriole
b) Vasa recta
c) Peritubular capillary
d) Interlobular vein

72. **Blood vessels that surround loops of Henle are**

a) Vasa recta
b) Peritubular capillaries
c) Interlobular arteries
d) Efferent arterioles

73. **Process that is most affected by blood pressure is**

a) Tubular secretion
b) Tubular reabsorption
c) Glomerular filtration
d) Loop of Henle diffusion

74. **Which of the following is not found in glomerular filtrate**

a) Glucose
b) Protein
c) Uric acid
d) Creatinine

75. **Muscle metabolism waste product that is eliminated by kidney is**

a) Urea b) Uric acid
c) Creatine d) Creatinine

76. **What is highest concentration in urine**

a) Glucose b) Sodium
c) Uric acid d) Phosphate

77. **Which ion is reabsorbed in exchange for sodium**

a) Chloride b) Potassium
c) Calcium d) Magnesium

78. **What is the average glomerular filtration rate per day**

a) 10-20L b) 180-200L
c) 1500-2000 ml d) 1000-5000 ml

79. **Which of the following is usually not found in urine**

a) Magnesium b) Urea
c) Uric acid d) Glucose

80. **How much urine is formed in 24 hours**

a) 12 liters b) 100 ml
c) 1.5 L d) 3 L

81. **Renin acts on ________ to convert it to angiotensin-I**

a) Angiotensin II b) Angiotensinogen
c) ACE d) Aldosterone

82. **The targets of angiotensin- II are blood vessels and ________**

a) Nerves b) Adrenal cortex
c) Adrenal medulla d) kidney nephron

83. **Tubular reabsorption occurs from the nephron tubules into the**

a) Loop of Henle b) Peritubular capillaries
c) Renal corpuscle d) Renal pyramid

84. Most tubular reabsorption occurs at the

a) Loop of Henle
b) Distal convoluted tubule
c) Proximal convoluted tubule
d) Glomerulus

85. Where are most microvilli found

a) Loop of Henle
b) Distal convoluted tubule
c) Vasa recta
d) Proximal convoluted tubule

86. What occurred by active transport

a) Excretion of albumin in the urine
b) Excretion of creatine in the urine
c) Reabsorption of water at the proximal tubule
d) Reabsorption of amino acids

87. Which one does not operate under a renal threshold mechanism

a) Creatine
b) Ascorbic acid
c) Sodium
d) Citric acid

88. Action of aldosterone is to increase

a) Sodium elimination
b) Sodium reabsorption
c) Potassium reabsorption
d) Chloride excretion

89. How much sodium is actively reabsorbed by the proximal segment of the nephron

a) 10%
b) 1%
c) 70%
d) 99%

90. Countercurrent multiplier mechanism occurs at

a) Proximal convoluted tubule
b) Loop of Henle
c) Distal convoluted tubule
d) Collecting ducts

91. Fluid in descending limb of loop of henle is ________ compare to capillaries

a) Isotonic
b) Weakly hypotonic
c) Strongly hypotonic
d) Hypertonic

92. Function of countercurrent multiplier is to

a) Increase the concentration of NaCl
b) Decrease the concentration of NaCl
c) Change the blood levels of potassium
d) Conserve potassium

93. ADH cause ________ in urine output

a) Minimal
b) Increases
c) Decreases
d) Maintains

94. ADH have greatest effect on

a) Loop of Henle
b) Proximal convoluted tubule
c) Distal convoluted tubule
d) Glomerulus

95. Large amounts of meat eating increase ________ in the blood

a) Protein
b) Creatinine
c) Urea
d) Uric acid

96. Uric acid results from ________ metabolism

a) Protein
b) Carbohydrate
c) Purine
d) Pyrimidine

97. Renal secretion of a compound occurs from ________ to the distal convoluted tubule

a) Loop of Henle
b) Glomerulus
c) Vasa recta
d) Peritubular capillaries

98. Which of these is not secreted by kidneys

a) Creatine
b) Creatinine
c) H+
d) Penicillin

99. Compound which is used to assess the function of kidney at level of glomerulus is

a) Creatinine
b) Inulin
c) Para-aminohippuric acid
d) Creatine

100. Which appears in urine as of dieting or excess utilization of lipids

a) Urea
b) Uric acid
c) Glycine
d) Ketone

101. Heavy exercise could release high amounts of ________ in urine

a) Glucose b) Uric acid
c) Albumin d) Ascorbic acid

102. What causes urine to flow from the kidneys to the bladder

a) Gravity b) Hydrostatic pressure
c) Peristalsis d) Osmotic pressure

103. Renal calculi are usually comprised of the following except

a) Calcium oxalate b) Cholesterol
c) Uric acid d) Magnesium phosphate

104. Mucosa of bladder is comprised of ________

a) Smooth muscle b) Squamous epithelium
c) Transitional epithelium d) Simple columnar epithelium

105. Which of these is under voluntary control

a) Urethra b) Detrusor muscle
c) Internal sphincter d) External sphincter

106. Micturition reflex is centered in

a) Medulla b) Sacral cord
c) Hypothalamus d) Lumbar cord

107. Statement that does not correctly characterize the kidney

a) Kidneys are positioned retroperitoneally
b) Right kidney is usually 1.5 to 2 centimeters higher than the left one
c) Kidney is padded by a layer of fat
d) Inside the kidney there is a hollow chamber called the renal sinus

108. Granular appearance of the renal cortex is due to

a) Positioning of blood vessels within this area
b) Polycystic kidney disease
c) Random distribution of nephrons in this area
d) Positioning of the renal columns

109. Which of these is not a function of kidney

a) Kidneys deactivate vitamin D and stimulate the activity of osteoclasts
b) Kidneys help control the rate of red blood cell production
c) Kidneys help to regulate blood pressure
d) Kidneys regulate the composition, volume and pH of body fluids

110. Final branches of interlobular arteries give rise to ________ that carry blood to the nephrons

a) Interlobar arteries b) Arciform arteries
c) Efferent arterioles d) Afferent arterioles

111. Trait that does not characterize the structure of a nephron

a) There are two coiled portions of the renal tubule
b) Glomerular capsule contains podocytes and slit pores
c) Blood that will be filtered flows into the glomerular capsule
d) Several nephron tubules merge to form a collecting duct

112. Which force favors filtration

a) Glomerular capillary hydrostatic pressure
b) Capsular hydrostatic pressure
c) Glomerular capillary osmotic pressure
d) Capsular osmotic pressure

113. Which factor does not affect glomerular filtration rate

a) Blood pressure
b) Osmotic pressure of the glomerular filtrate
c) Plasma osmotic pressure
d) Concentration of leukocytes in the blood

114. Juxtaglomerular cells of kidney secrete ________ when blood pressure drops

a) Angiotensin b) Potassium
c) Renin d) Atrial natriuretic peptide

115. Where does most selective reabsorption occur

a) Loop of Henle b) Glomerulus
c) Distal convoluted tubule d) Proximal convoluted tubule

116. How afferent arteriole differ in size from efferent arteriole

a) Afferent arteriole is longer
b) Afferent arteriole has larger diameter
c) Afferent arteriole is rounder
d) Afferent arteriole has smaller diameter

117. Urine formation requires

a) Glomerular filtration and tubular secretion only
b) Glomerular filtration and tubular reabsorption only
c) Glomerular filtration, tubular reabsorption, and tubular secretion
d) Tubular reabsorption and secretion only

118. Which of the following is not a normal filtrate component

a) Large proteins b) Glucose
c) Nitrogenous wastes d) Amino acids

119. When osmolality of the blood increases

a) ADH secretion is decreased
b) Blood volume increase
c) Both occur
d) Neither occur

120. Increase in sodium reabsorption in distal convoluted tubules is due to

a) Increase in the production of aldosterone
b) Increase in the production of ADH
c) Increase in osmolarity of blood plasma
d) Increase in the production of Oxytocin

121. Ability of the kidney is to produce either hyperosmotic or hyposmotic urine depends in part on

a) Amount of hydrogen ion and ammonium ion secreted
b) Afferent and efferent arteriole relationship
c) Absorbing ability of the collecting tubule
d) Counter current multiplier mechanism of loop of Henle

122. If there is high level of creatinine in blood, this could be assumed of

a) Urinary tract infection b) Diabetes
c) Kidney failure d) Normal condition

123. Direct control of water excretion in kidneys is controlled by

a) Anti-diuretic hormone
b) Oxytocin
c) Blood plasma
d) Sodium amounts in the blood

124. Nephrons helps in

a) Eliminate wastes from the body
b) Regulate blood volume and pressure
c) Control levels of electrolytes and metabolites
d) Regulate blood pH
e) All of the above

125. If an animal is dehydrated, his body will increase

a) ATP
b) ADP
c) Diluted urine
d) ADH

126. Which part of the nephron removes water, ions and nutrients from blood

a) Vasa recta
b) Loop of henle
c) Glomerulus
d) Peritubular capillaries

127. Kidneys have a direct effect on

a) Blood pressure
b) Total blood volume
c) pH
d) All of the above

128. Why substances in the glomerulus enter Bowman's capsule

a) Magnetic charge of the Bowman's capsule attracts the substances
b) Substances are actively transported into the Bowman's capsule
c) Blood pressure of glomerulus is so great that most substances in blood move into capsule
d) None

129. In tubular excretion

a) Urine bonds are formed between wastes
b) Wastes are diffused from tubule
c) Wastes move into distal convoluted tubule from blood
d) Blood pressure forces wastes away from kidney

130. Countercurrent exchange system includes _____ and _____.

a) Glomerulus and macula densa
b) Proximal convoluted tubule and distal convoluted tubule
c) Loop of Henle and Vasa recta
d) Afferent arteriole and efferent arteriole

131. Function of the loop of henle in process of urine formation is

a) Reabsorption of water
b) Production of filtrate
c) Reabsorption of solutes
d) Secretion of solutes

132. Function of the macula densa cells is to

a) Prevent water reabsorption in ascending loop of Henle
b) Add bicarbonate ions to the tubular Filtrate
c) Secrete renin in response to decreased afferent arteriole pressure
d) Monitor NaCl concentration in filtrate

133. Atrial naturiuretic peptide works to

a) Increase afferent arteriole pressure
b) Increase blood flow to kidney
c) Enhance the effects of ADH
d) Inhibit effects of aldosterone

134. If level of aldosterone in blood increases, then

a) Less sodium is excreted in urine
b) Less potassium is excreted in urine
c) Systemic blood pressure will decrease
d) Glomerular filtration will decrease

135. Most important function of juxtaglomerular apparatus is to

a) Secrete water and sodium into filtrate
b) Reabsorb sodium
c) Generate bicarbonate ions in response to decreased blood pH
d) Secrete renin in response to decreased renal blood pressure or blood flow

136. If diameter of afferent arteriole is smaller than diameter of the efferent arteriole, then

a) Net filtration pressure will decrease
b) Blood pressure in the glomerulus will decrease
c) GFR will increase
d) a and b

137. From distal convoluted tubule, filtrate is carried to

a) Renal corpuscle
b) Collecting duct
c) Nephron loop
d) Proximal convoluted tubule

138. A dog who is dehydrated from vomition and diarrhea, blood will have higher in

a) ADH
b) Aldosterone
c) Both ADH and aldosterone
d) None

139. All of the following are normally found in urine except

a) Glucose
b) Sodium ions
c) Uric acid
d) Urea

140. Which region of the nephron contains capillaries

a) Renal glomerulus
b) Proximal convoluted tubule
c) Nephron loop
d) Distal tubule

141. Angiotensin I is ________ aminoacid peptide

a) 6
b) 8
c) 10
d) 12

142. Modern theory of urine formation was proposed by

a) Arthur Cushney
b) William Bowman
c) Claudius Galen
d) Carl Ludwig

143. Rate at which blood flows to the kidney is called

a) Renal blood flow
b) Filtration fraction
c) Glomerular Filtration Rate
d) All

144. Counter current multiplier mechanism occurs in

a) Vasa Recta b) Bowmans capsule
c) Loops of Henle d) Juxta glomerular apparatus

145. Ammonia is converted to Uric acid in which part of birds

a) Liver b) Kidney
c) Cloaca d) Liver and Kidney both

146. The principal nitrogenous component of avian urine is

a) Ammonia b) Urea
c) Uric acid d) Amino acid

147. Which one of the following nephron component is lacking in Reptilian nephron

a) Proximal tubule b) Loop of Henle
c) Distal tubule d) Collecting duct

Answer

1. c	2. b	3. c	4. c	5. b	6. d	7. d	8. d	9. c	10. c
11. c	12. d	13. b	14. d	15. b	16. b	17. d	18. c	19. d	20. d
21. b	22. d	23. d	24. a	25. d	26. a	27. d	28. b	29. d	30. a
31. c	32. c	33. d	34. e	35. a	36. b	37. a	38. b	39. d	40. b
41. c	42. d	43. b	44. a	45. d	46. c	47. b	48. b	49. c	50. a
51. d	52. a	53. b	54. d	55. d	56. c	57. b	58. a	59. c	60. b
61. d	62. c	63. b	64. d	65. b	66. a	67. b	68. c	69. a	70. c
71. d	72. a	73. c	74. b	75. d	76. b	77. b	78. b	79. d	80. c
81. b	82. b	83. b	84. c	85. d	86. d	87. c	88. b	89. c	90. b
91. d	92. a	93. c	94. c	95. c	96. c	97. d	98. a	99. b	100. d
101. c	102. c	103. b	104. c	105. d	106. b	107. b	108. c	109. a	110. d
111. c	112. a	113. d	114. c	115. d	116. b	117. c	118. a	119. b	120. a
121. d	122. c	123. a	124. e	125. d	126. d	127. d	128. c	129. c	130. c
131. a	132. d	133. d	134. a	135. d	136. d	137. b	138. d	139. a	140. a
141. c	142. a	143. a	144. c	145. d	146. c	147. b			

□□□

CHAPTER-9

Muscular System

All skeletal muscle is consists of numerous multinucleated fibers. This muscle fiber contain several myofibrils, each myofibril is composed of 1500 myosin filaments and 3000 actin filaments. These actin and myosin are protein molecules and responsible for muscle contraction. The myosin filament is called **thick filaments** and actin filament is called **thin filaments**. The light bands contain only actin filament and are called I bands or Isotropic to polarized light, where as myosin is anisotropic to polarized light and called A bands. Entire muscle fibre has light and dark bands which gives both skeletal and cardiac muscle a **striated appearance**. Myfibrils are suspended inside muscle fiber in an intracellular matrix (cytoplasm) called **sarcoplasm.**

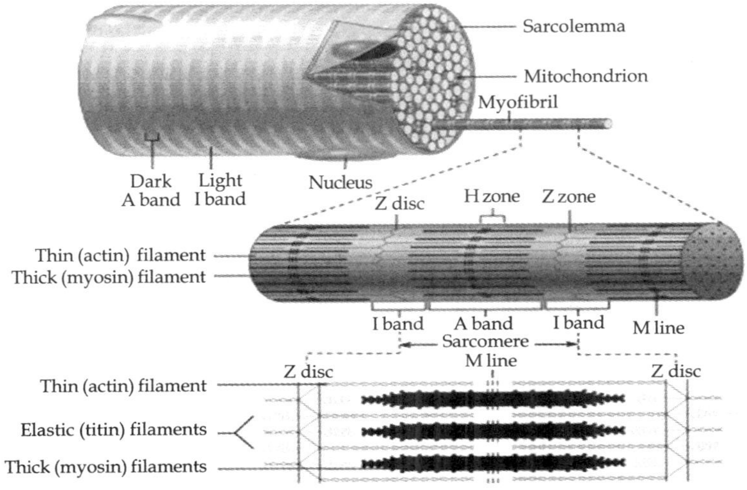

Microscopic structure of skeletal muscle

Neuromuscular Junction

Each nerve ending makes a junction with the muscle fiber called **Neuromuscular Junction**. The branches of nerve fiber at its end form a complex which invaginates into muscle fiber but lie outside the muscle fiber plasma membrane. This entire structure is called **motor end plate**. The space between the axon terminal and the muscle fiber membrane is called **synaptic space or synaptic cleft**. Acetyl choline is neuro-transmitter in neuromuscular junction that helps in transmission of impulse. Muscle contraction occurs by sliding filament mechanism where actin filaments slide inward among myosin filaments. This sliding mechanism is caused by the mechanical forces generated by interaction of the crossbridges of myosin filaments with actin filaments. This mechanical forces is produced by the Ca+ ion release from sarcoplasmic reticulum as of action potential travels over the muscle fiber. Myosin filament is composed of multiple myosin molecule. It is composed of 6 polypeptide chains, two heavy chains and four light chains. Actin filament is a complex protein and composed of 3 protein components as actin, tropomyosin and troponin. Each **troponin molecule is a** complex of 3 loosely bound protein subunits as **troponin I** which has affinity for actin, **troponin T** which has affinity for tropomyosin and troponin C which has affinity for calcium. This complex is believed to attach the tropomyosin to actin. The strong affinity of troponin for calcium ion is believed to initiate the contraction process. Phosphocreatine in muscle is the major sources of energy for muscle contraction. When total mass of muscle enlarge it is called Muscle Hypertrophy but when decreases is called Atrophy. Muscle hypertrophy results by increasing in the number of actin and myosin filaments in each muscle fiber. Condition where the number of muscle fibers increases is called fiber hyperplasia. Several hours after death all the muscles of the body goes into a state of contracture called **Rigor mortis**. This rigidity is caused by loss of all ATPs which are required to cause separation off the cross bridges from the actin filaments during relaxation process.

Smooth muscle is present in blood vessels, GI tract and urinary bladder etc. It is composed of far smaller fibers which are elongated and thin that contain single nucleus. Smooth muscle contain actin and myosin but these proteins are more loosely organized than they are in skeletal and cardiac muscles and don't form myofibrils so not striated. Sarcomere, Troponin and T-tubules are absent in smooth muscle. Contraction of smooth muscle is prolonged some times last even hrs or day but contraction of skeletal muscle is faster. There are two major types of smooth muscle as multiunit smooth muscle and unitary (single unit) smooth muscle. In smooth muscle large number of actin filaments are attached called dense bodies. Where as myosin filaments interspersed among many actin filaments. In place of troponin smooth muscle contain large amount of protein similar to troponin called **calmodulin**. Camodulin-calcium complex activate myosine kinase which phosphorylate light chain (regulatory chain) of myosine head as of which the head of myosine has capability to bind with actin filament and cause contraction in same way as skeletal muscle. Although skeletal muscle fiber are activated exclusively by nervous system but smooth muscle can be stimulated by multiple types of signals like hormonal, neural, receptor proteins which also initiates contractile process.

Cardiac Muscle is striated in structure as skeletal muscle. T-tubules are larger in cardiac muscle than skeletal muscle. It has the typical myofibril that contain Actin and Myosin filaments almost identical to those in skeletal muscle. But there are otherways by which cardiac muscles are different from skeletal muscles. The cell of cardiac muscle is single nucleated. The dark areas crossing the cardiac muscle fibers are called **intercalated discs**. They are actually cell membranes that separate individual cardiac muscle cells from one another. The cardiac cells are so interconnected that when one of the cell become excited the action potential spreads to all of them spreading from cell to cell throughout the interconnections. So cardiac muscle is a syncytium. The heart is composed of two syncitium as atrial syncitium and ventricular syncitium.

Membrane Potential is the potential difference between outer and inner membrane fiber. To measure the membrane potential microtodes are used. Out side of the membrane is positive where as inside of the membrane is negative. The resting membrane potential of skeletal fiber is -90 mv where as membrane potential of smooth muscle is -50 to -60mV which is 30mV less negative to skeletal muscle. In skeletal muscle Signals are transmitted by action potential which are rapid changes in membrane potential that spreads rapidly along the fiber membrane. Each action potential begins with sudden change from the normal negative membrane potential to a positive potential then ends with equal negative potential. It can also be defined as the rapid change in polarity that moves along the muscle fiber is called the **action Potential.** Successive stages of action Potential are resting Stage or polarised stage, depolarised stage and repolarized stage. Action potential occurs in unitary smooth muscle not in multi unit smooth muscle. The action potential in unitary smooth muscle are in two forms as **spike potential** and **action potential with plateau**. Action potential in cardiac muscle goes upto +20mV from a negative membrane potential of -85mV. But after initial spike the membrane remain depolarized for about 0.2 second in atrial muscle and about 0.3 second in ventricular muscle exhibiting a **plateau** followed at the end of the plateau by abrupt (sudden) repolarization. The presence of this plateau in the action potential cause muscle contraction to last upto 15 times as long in cardiac muscle than skeletal muscle.

Short Questions and Answers

1. What is anatomy of Skeletal muscle?

Ans. All skeletal muscle is consists of numerous multinucleated fibers which are of 10-80 μm in diameter. This muscle fiber contain several myofibrils, each myofibril is composed of 1500 myosin filaments and 3000 actin filaments. These actin and myosin are protein molecules and responsible for muscle contraction. The myoin are thick called **thick filaments** and actin are thin called **thin filaments**. The light bands contain only actin filament and are called I bands or Isotropic to polarized light, where as myosin is anisotropic to polarized light and called A bands. Therefore the entire muscle fibre has light and dark bands which gives both skeletal and cardiac muscle a **striated appearance**. At the end of the actin filament another protein is attached called Z-disc. The portion of myofibril that lies between two successive Z-disc is called **sarcomere.** When the muscle fiber is at normal the length of sarcomere is about 2 μm. At this length actin filament overlap the myosin filament and the sarcomere at this length is also capable of generating its greatest force of contraction.

2. How impulse transmitted from nerves to skeletal muscle fiber?

Ans. The skeletal muscle fibers are inervated by large mylinated nerve fibers that are originated from spinal cord. Each nerve fiber after entering the muscle normally branches and stimulates several muscle fibers. Each nerve ending makes a junction with the muscle fiber called **neuromuscular Junction**.

The branches of nerve fiber at its end form a complex which invaginate into muscle fiber but lie outside the muscle fiber plasma membrane. This entire structure is called **motor end plate**. The invaginated axon terminal of neuron to muscle fiber is called **synaptic gutter or synaptic trough**. The space between the axon terminal and the muscle fiber membrane is called **synaptic space or synaptic cleft**. This space is about 20-30 nm wide. At the bottom of the synaptic gutter there are numerous smaller folds of the muscle membrane is called sub neural clefts. In the axon terminal mitochondria, ATP is used as energy source mainly for synthesis of excitatory transmitter, Ach. This Ach excites the muscle fiber. When nerve impulse reaches the neuromuscular junction , Ach is released from nerve terminal to synaptic space. This Ach binds to the Ach receptor present in the muscle membrane and cause opening of Ach-gated channels as of which large quantity of Na^+ ions passed into the interior of the fiber. This passage of Na^+ ions creates a local positive potential change inside the muscle membrane fiber called **end Plate Potential**. In turn this end plate potential spreading along the muscle membrane and cause muscle contraction.

3. What is myasthenia gravis?

Ans. It occurs about 1 in every 2000 persons which cause paralysis as of inability of the neuromuscular junction to transmit signals from nerve fiber to muscle fiber. In this condition antibodies that attack the Ach-gated Na^+ ion transport protein is seen in blood. Therefore it is believed that patient with myasthenia gravis is an autoimmune disease where patient develops immunity against their own Ach-activated ion channels, as of which the endplate potential that occur in muscle fiber are too weak to stimulate the fibers.

4. What is the general mechanism of skeletal muscle contraction?

Ans. Action potential don't occur spontaneously in skeletal muscle, they are produced in response to action potential in nerve fiber (Motor neuron). When an action potential travels along motor nerve to its ending on muscle fiber then nerve secretes a small amount of neurotransmitter called acetyl Choline

(Ach). Ach acts on muscle fiber to open Ach-gated channels in the membrane. Opening of Ach-gated channels allows large quantities of Na^+ ion flow in to the interior of the muscle fiber membrane. This initiates action potential in muscle fiber. The action potential depolarizes the muscle membrane and cause sarcoplasmic reticulum to release large quantities of calcium ion. Calcium initiates attractive force between Actin and Myosin filaments. After attraction of second, the Calcium ions pumped back to sarcoplasmic reticulum which cause muscle contraction to cease.

5. What is the structure of myosin filament?

Ans. Myosine filament is composed of multiple myosin molecule (around 200 or more), each having molecular weight of 480,000. It is composed of 6 polypeptide chains, two heavy chains (Each of MW of 200,000) and four light chains (each of 20,000). The two heavy chains wrap spirally around each other to form double helix called tail of the myosin. One end of these tail is folded in to globular polypeptide structure called myosin head. The four light chains are also the part of myosin head. Since myosin filament is consists of 200 or more myosin molecules, tail of all myosin molecules bundled together and form body of the filament. While the head of these molecules hangs together called cross-bridge. The total length of myosin filament is of 1.6μm long.

6. What is the structure of actin filament?

Ans. It is a complex protein and composed of 3 protein components as **actin, tropomyosin** and **troponin**. Each actin filament is of 1 μm long. Back bone of actin filament is a double helix **F-actin** protein molecule. This two F-actin molecule wound in a helix. And two strands of myosine molecule fits in the groove formed between the actin strand. Each tropomyosin molecule has mw 70,000 and length 40nm. These molecules wrap spirally around the sides of the F-actin helix. **Troponin molecule** is complex of 3 loosely bound protein subunits as **Troponin I** which has affinity for actin, **Troponin T** which has affinity for tropomyosin and **Troponin C** which has affinity for calcium. This troponin molecule complex is believed to attach the tropomyosin to actin. The strong affinity of troponin for calcium ion is believed to initiate the contraction process.

7. **What is membrane potential and action potential?**

Ans. **Membrane Potential** is the potential difference between outer and inner membrane fiber. To measure the membrane potential microtodes are used. Out side of the membrane is positive where as inside of the membrane is negative. The resting membrane potential of skeletal muscle fiber is -90 mV. Potential inside fiber is 90 mV more negative than the potential in the extra cellular fluid on the out side of the fiber. Nerve signals are transmitted by **action potential** which are rapid change in the membrane potential that spreads rapidly along the muscle fiber membrane. Each action potential begins with sudden change from the normal negative membrane potential to a positive potential then ends with equal negative potential. It can also be defined as the rapid change in polarity that moves along the muscle fiber is called the **Action Potential.** Successive stages of action potential are i) **resting stage** which is resting membrane potential before the action potential begins. During resting stage membrane is called **polarised stage** of -90mV, ii) d**epolarised stage:** at this stage membrane become suddenly permeable to Na+ ions and allows tremendous Na+ ions flow to interior of axon so the inside negative potential rise rapidly towards positive direction called depolarized stage, iii) **repolarized stage:** Within 10000th of a second after the membrane potential highly permeably to Na+ ions, the Na+ channels begins to close and the K+ channels open, then rapidly there is diffusion of K+ to the exterior part which establish normal negative resting membrane potential called repolarization of membrane.

8. **What is all or nothing principle?**

Ans. Once the action potential has been elicited at any point on the membrane of a normal fiber, the depolarization process travels over the entire membrane if conditions are right or it might not travel at all if conditions are not right. This is called **all or nothing principle**.

9. What is safety factor for propagation?

Ans. Some times the action potential reaches a point on the membrane at which it does not generate sufficient voltage to stimulate the next area of the membrane. When this occur the spread of depolarization stops. Therefore for continued propagation of an impulse to occur, the ratio of action potential to threshold for excitation must be greater than 1 at all times. This greater than 1 requirement is called **safety factor for propagation**.

10. What is absolute refractory period?

Ans. The period during which a second action potential can not be elicited even though a strong stimulus is applied is called **absolute refractory period**. This period for large nerve fiber is 1/250 sec and 0.25 to 0.30 for ventricle of heart. It may be otherwise defined as the brief period during which the muscle is not excitable to second stimulus is called **refractory period.**

11. What are the sources of energy for muscle contraction?

Ans. Muscle contraction depends upon the energy supplied by ATP. There are several sources of energy for this rephosphorylation. These sources of energy are i) **Phosphocreatine in muscle:** Phosphocreatine carries high energy phosphate bonds. This bond instantly cleaved and release energy cause bonding of new phosphate ion to ADP to reconstitute the ATP, ii) **Glycogen stored in muscle:** Rapidly breakdown of glycogen to pyruvic acid and lactic acid liberate energy that is used to convert ADP to ATP and iii) **Oxidative metabolism:** This is the third source of energy and it means combining of oxygen with various cellular food stuffs to liberate energy. These food stuffs are carbohydrate, protein and Fat.

12. What is isometric and isotonic contraction?

Ans. Muscle contraction is said to be **isometric** when muscle does not shorten during contraction and when muscle is shorten with the tension on the muscle remains constant is called **isotonic contraction.**

13. What is excitation contraction coupling? or How action potential passes interior of the muscle fiber?

Ans. The skeletal muscle fiber is so long that the action potential spreading along its surface membrane cause almost no current flow deep within the fiber. However to muscle contraction, these electrical currents must penetrate deeply in to the muscle fiber. This is only achieved by transmission of action potential along **transverse tubules (T tubules)** that penetrate all the way through the muscle fiber from one side of muscle fiber to other. The action potential in T-tubules cause release of ca^{+2} ions in the immediate vicinity of all myofibrils and cause contraction. This total process is called **excitation contraction coupling**. The T-tubules are very small and run transverse to the myofibril. They begin at the cell membrane and penetrate all the way from one side of the muscle fiber to opposite side. Therefore when action potential spreads over muscle fiber membrane, a potential change also spreads along T-tubules to the deep interior of the muscle fiber. As of this action potential there is release of ca^{+2} ion from sarcoplasmic reticulum, which binds strongly with troponin C and cause entire muscle contraction.

14. What is rigor mortis?

Ans. Several hours after death all the muscles of the body goes into a state of contracture called **rigor mortis**. That is muscle contract and become rigid even without action potential. This rigidity is caused by loss of all ATPs which are required to cause separation off the cross bridges from the actin filaments during relaxation process. The muscle remain in the riger until the muscle proteins are destroyed, which usually results from autolysis caused by enzyme release from lysosomes 15-25 hr later.

15. What is the mechanism of smooth muscle contraction?

Ans. In place of troponin smooth muscle contain large amount of protein similar to troponin called **calmodulin**. Calcium releases from sarcoplasmic reticulum binds to calmodulin light chain of myosine head (1 calmodulin attach to 4 calcium). Camodulin-calcium complex activate myosine kinase which phosphorylate light chain (regulatory chain) of myosine head as of which the head of myosine has capability to bind with actin filament and cause contraction in same way as skeletal muscle.

16. What is membrane potential action potential of smooth muscle?

Ans. Membrane potential of smooth muscle is -50 to -60mV which is 30mV less negative to skeletal muscle. Action potential occurs in unitary smooth muscle (present in visceral muscle) not in multi unit smooth muscle. The action potential in unitary smooth muscle are in two forms as **spike potential and action potential with plateau**. **Spike potential** is seen in skeletal muscle occurs most of unitary smooth muscle. In **action potential with plateau** instead of rapid repolarization the muscle fiber membrane, the repolarization is delayed for several hundred to thousand milliseconds. The smooth muscle membrane has more voltage gated Ca^{+2} channels than voltage gated Na^+ channels. Therefore Na^+ participation is little in generation of action potential in smooth muscle. Instead flow of Ca^{+2} ions in interior of the fiber is mainly responsible for the action potential.

17. What is structure of cardiac muscle?

Ans. It is striated in structure as skeletal muscle. T-tubules are larger in cardiac muscle than skeletal muscle. It has the typical myofibril that contain actin and myosin filaments almost identical to those in skeletal muscle. But there are otherways by which cardiac muscles are different from skeletal muscles. The cell of cardiac muscle is single nucleated. The dark areas crossing the cardiac muscle fibers are called **intercalated discs**. They are actually cell membranes that separate individual cardiac muscle cells from one another. Cardiac muscle fibers are made up of mainly individual cells connected in series with one another. The cardiac cells are so interconnected that when one of the cell become excited the action potential spreads to all of them spreading from cell to cell throughout the interconnections. So cardiac muscle is a **syncytium**. The cell membrane of cardiac muscle fiber are fuse with one another in such a way that they form permeable communicating junctions called Gap Junctions that allows almost totally free diffusion of all ions. So the action potential travels from one cardiac muscle cell to the next. The heart is composed of two syncitium as atrial syncitium and ventricular syncitium.

18. What cause the long action potential and plateau in cardiac muscle?

Ans. This is because of two major differences between membrane properties of cardiac and skeletal muscle. They are as such

i) The action potential of skeletal muscle is caused entirely by sudden opening of large number of fast Sodium channels. These channels are called fast as it remains open for 10,000th of a second and then suddenly close but in cardiac muscle the action potential is caused by the opening of two types of channels. They are 1) Fast Na+ channel like in skeletal muscle 2) By slow Ca+2 channels called Calcium-Sodium channels. This slow Ca+2 channels differs from fast Na+ channels by slower to open and even remain open for several tenth of a second. During this time a large quantity of both calcium and sodium ions flow through these channels to the interior of the cardiac muscle fiber and this maintains a prolonged period of depolarization causing plateau in action potential. Furthermore the ca+2 ions that enter during this action potential plays an important role in helping to excite the muscle contractile process/ muscle contraction.

ii) The second major functional difference between cardiac and skeletal muscle for prolonged action potential and plateau is that immediately after onset of the action potential the permeability of cardiac muscle membrane for K+ ion decreases about 5 fold, the effect that does not occur in the skeletal muscle. This decreased K+ permeability may be caused by the excess Ca+2 influx through the Ca+2 channels. This decreased K+ permeability greatly decreases the outflux of K+ ions during the action potential plateau and there by prevents early return of action potential to its resting level.

19. What is muscle fatigue?

Ans. Muscle fatigue is the condition resulting from prolonged and strong contraction of muscle. If muscle is stimulated at a sufficient high rate to prevent relaxation between contraction a continuous contracted state developed called **titany**. This titany occurs because the calcium pumps of the sarccoplasmic membrane can not remove the cytoplasmic calcium as fast as it is released by the action potential. When muscle titany is maintained for a long time even though stimulation is continued this is called **muscle fatigue**.

20. What are the energy sources for muscle contraction?

Ans. There are two ways of energy sources for muscle contraction as aerobic metabolism and anaerobic metabolism

For aerobic metabolism oxygen goes in blood stream but during intense exercise there is deprivation of oxygen as of which anaerobic metabolism is activated which can only produce certain amount of energy at a time not over hours like aerobic metabolism. So during this anaerobic metabolism there is increase in concentration of **lactic acid** and hydrogen ion. During prolonged muscle fatigue there is depletion of muscle glycogen.

21. What is Trappe or Ascending staircase effect?

Ans. When skeletal muscle is stimulated to contract while still undergoing relaxation or during a period immediately after relaxation, a second muscle twitch is produced and develops a greater tension than the initial contraction. This is called **temporal summation** of muscle contraction. This temporal summation is best observed when the muscle is repetitively stimulated to produce series of contraction. Each subsequent contraction demonstrates an increase in tension over the previous contraction until a plateau of maximum tension is attained. This is called **Trappe or Ascending staircase effect.**

Choose the Best Answer

1. **Smooth Muscle is**

   a) Voluntary and Spindle Shaped
   b) Voluntary and Striated
   c) Involuntary and Spindle shaped
   d) Involuntary and Striated

2. **Skeletal Muscle is**

   a) Voluntary and Spindle Shaped
   b) Voluntary and Striated
   c) Involuntary and SpindleShaped
   d) Involuntary and Striated

3. **Cardiac Muscle is**

   a) Voluntary and Spindle Shaped
   b) Voluntary and Striated
   c) Involuntary and Spindle Shaped
   d) Involuntary and Striated

4. **Multinucleated muscle cell is**

   a) Cardiac b) Smooth
   c) Skeletal d) All of the Above

5. **Example of a smooth muscle is**

   a) Masseter b) Bladder
   c) Heart d) Rectus Abdominis

6. **Each myosin filament is surrounded by how many actin filaments**

   a) Two b) Four
   c) Six d) Eight

7. **Muscular system is controlled by**

   a) Cardiovascular system b) Integumentary System
   c) Nervous system d) None of the above

8. **How many types of muscle are there**

   a) Two b) Three
   c) Four d) Five

9. Skeletal muscle is described by all of the following except

a) Striated b) Voluntary
c) Multinucleate d) Autorhythmic

10. Walls of hollow organs and some blood vessels contain which muscle tissue

a) Striated b) Skeletal
c) Cardiac d) Smooth

11. Cardiac muscle tissue is unique because of

a) Involuntary action b) Non-striated appearance
c) Intercalated discs d) Containing smooth muscle tissue

12. Approximately what percentage of body heat is generated by muscle tissue

a) 15% b) 30%
c) 55% d) 85%

13. A muscle fascicle is a

a) Bundle of myofibrils b) Bundle of connective tissue
c) Bundle of muscle fibers d) Muscle cell

14. Smallest contractile unit of skeletal muscle is

a) Sarcomere b) Motor unit
c) Synapse d) Thin filament

15. Major regulatory proteins in muscle tissue are

a) Myosin and Tropomyosin b) Myosin and Actin
c) Actin and Troponin d) Troponin and Tropomyosin

16. Which of the actions is caused by skeletal muscle

a) Heartbeat b) Constriction of blood vessels
c) Dilation of pupil d) Eye movements

17. Which of the following does not occur during muscle contraction

a) Thick and thin filaments bind to each other
b) Muscle fibers stretch
c) Thick and thin filaments slide each other
d) Muscle fibers shorten

18. Process aids in skeletal muscle relaxation after contraction

a) Calcium is released from intracellular storage sites
b) Motor neurons send electrical signal to muscle
c) Acetylcholinesterease degrades acetylcholine
d) Troponin binds calcium

19. Stiffness of muscle tissue in rigor mortis partially results from

a) Excessive acetycholine activity on muscle
b) Excessive calcium release in muscle
c) Excessive lactic acid build up
d) Excessive contraction of the fibers

20. Hormone that stimulates the breakdown of bone and the increase in blood calcium levels

a) Growth hormone
b) Estrogen
c) Parathyroid hormone
d) Calcitonin

21. When an action potential reaches the presynaptic terminal of the motor neuron

a) Calcium is released inside of the muscle fiber
b) Acetylcholine is released into the synaptic cleft
c) Acetylcholinesterease is released into synaptic cleft
d) Physical contact between the motor neuron and the muscle fiber occurs

22. Lack of acetylcholinesterase in the synaptic cleft would result in

a) Decrease acetylcholine production by motor neuron
b) Relaxation of the muscle fiber
c) Excessive, continuous stimulation of muscle fiber
d) Inability of the motor neuron to stimulate muscle fiber

23. Toxin thst blocks the acetylcholine receptors on muscle tissue result in

a) Increased stimulation of the muscle fiber
b) Inability of the muscle to respond to motor nerve stimulus
c) Contraction of the muscle fiber
d) Excessive contractions and convulsions

24. Exercises causes

a) Increase number of mitochondria per muscle fiber
b) Increase number of muscle fibers
c) Increase number of motor units
d) Increase number of skeletal muscles

25. Muscular dystrophy is a congenital disorder that is characterized by

a) Skeletal muscle degeneration
b) Excessive convulsion
c) Shaking and trembling
d) Only cardiac damage

26. Which disorders is characterized by painful musculoskeletal "tender points"

a) Fibromyalgia
b) Myasthenia gravis
c) Duchenne muscular dystrophy
d) Becker muscular dystrophy

27. Anabolic steroids have all effects except

a) Builds muscle proteins
b) Increases muscle strength
c) Increases number of muscles in body
d) Result in liver cancer and heart disease

28. Which statements regarding aging and muscular system is true

a) Aging is associated with decreased myoglobin production
b) Effects of aging can be nearly completely reversed
c) Satellite cells increase in aging causing fibrosis
d) Young persons have more adipose in muscles compared to elderly persons

29. Dense connective tissue covering outer surface of bone diaphyses is termed

a) Perichondrium b) Periosteum
c) Endosteum d) Exofibrium

30. Hormone that promotes glucose and amino acid uptake by muscle

a) Adrenaline
b) Insulin
c) Glucagon
d) Cortisol

31. Which two components in bone are responsible for hardness and pliability of bone

a) Osteoclasts & Collagen
b) Mineralized salts & Osteocytes
c) Mineralized salts & Collagen
d) Collagen & Elastic fibers

32. Glucose enters muscle cells mostly by

a) Simple diffusion
b) Facilitated diffusion using a specific glucose transporter
c) Co-transport with sodium
d) Co-transport with amino acids

33. Yellow marrow consists of

a) Osteoprogenitor cells
b) Blood cell progenitor cells
c) Hyaline cartilage
d) Adipose

34. Chondroblasts produce

a) Basement membranes
b) Bone matrix
c) Cartilage matrix
d) Mesothelium

35. Structures that are at the center of compact bone lamellae and carry blood vessels along the bone length

a) Haversian canals
b) Canaliculi
c) Perforating canals
d) Osteocytes

36. Cell type that is responsible for maintaining bone matrix once formed is

a) Osteoclasts
b) Osteoblasts
c) Osteocytes
d) Fibroblasts

37. Glycogen breakdown in exercising muscle is activated by

a) Insulin
b) Cortisol
c) Amylase
d) None of the above

38. Type I muscle fibres is

a) White, glycolytic, slow contracting
b) White, oxidative, slow contracting
c) Red, glycolytic, slow contracting
d) Red, oxidative, slow contracting

39. Two principal contractile proteins in skeletal muscle are

a) Actin and troponin
b) Actin and myosin
c) Troponin and tropomyosin
d) Myosin and tropomyosin

40. Sarcoplasmic reticulum in muscle cells acts as

a) Store of digestive enzymes
b) Store of sodium ions
c) Store of lipid
d) Store of calcium ions

41. An action potential arriving at the motor endplate causes release of

a) Acetylcholine which traverses the neuromuscular junction
b) Sodium ions which binds to sodium receptors on the muscle membrane
c) Calcium ions which initiate an action potential along the muscle fibre
d) Noradrenaline which increases muscle metabolic activity

42. The trigger to initiate the contractile process in skeletal muscle is

a) Potassium binding to myosin
b) Calcium binding to tropomyosin
c) ATP binding to the myosin cross bridges
d) Calcium binding to troponin

43. After calcium ions have been released from the sarcoplasmic reticulum they

a) Initiate an action potential
b) Cause sodium channels to open in the sarcolemmal membrane
c) Bind to troponin
d) Bind to actin

44. Muscle fibre relaxes when

a) Nerve stimulus is removed
b) Nerve stimulus is too forceful
c) Actin binding sites are uncovered
d) Actin binding sites are saturated

45. Fast-twitch fibres contain

a) Large number of mitochondria and low ATPase activity
b) Small number of mitochondria and low ATPase activity
c) Small number of mitochondria and high ATPase activity
d) Large number of mitochondria and high ATPase activity

46. Muscle protein acts as ATPase is

a) Actin
b) Myosine
c) Both
d) None

47. Inter calated disc are present in

a) Skeletal muscle fiber
b) Smooth muscle fiber
c) Cardiac muscle fiber
d) All

48. Distance between two Z-line in skeletal muscle fiber is called

a) Sarcolemma
b) Sarcomere
c) Titin
d) None

49. During muscle contraction size of I band

a) Decrease
b) Increase
c) Remain constant
d) None

50. Major protein in thick filament of skeletal muscle fiber is

a) Actin
b) Myosine
c) Both
d) None

51. Major protein in thin filament of skeletal muscle fiber is

a) Actin
b) Myosine
c) Both
d) None

52. Fundamental repeating unit of a skeletal muscle fiber is

a) Sarcolemma
b) Sarcomere
c) Actin
d) Myosine

53. Ion which is essential for muscle contraction is

a) Na^{+} b) K^{+}
c) Ca^{+2} d) Mg^{+2}

54. Immediate source of energy for muscle contraction is

a) Glucose b) Creatine phosphate
c) Glycogen d) ATP

55. Muscle contraction is said to be isometric when

a) Muscle does not shorten during contraction
b) Muscle shorten during contraction.
c) Either a or b
d) Both a & b

56. Muscle contraction is said to be isotonic when

a) Muscle does not shorten during contraction
b) Muscle shorten during contraction with the tension on the muscle remains constant
c) Either a or b
d) Both a & b

57. Invaginated axon terminal of neuron to muscle fiber in neuro muscular junction is called

a) Synaptic gutter b) Synaptic trough
c) Synaptic cleft d) Both a & b

58. Space between axon terminal and the muscle fiber membrane in neuro muscular junction is called

a) Synaptic gutter
b) Synaptic cleft or Synaptic space
c) Synaptic trough
d) All

59. Myosin filaments are called

a) Thick filament b) Thin filament
c) Both d) None

60. Actin are thin called

a) Thick filament b) Thin filament
c) Both d) None

61. The portion of myofibril that lies between two successive Z-disc of skeletal muscle is called

a) Sarcolemma
b) Sarcomere
c) Sarcoplasm
d) All

62. Membrane of muscle fiber is

a) Sarcolemma
b) Sarcomere
c) Sarcoplasm
d) All

63. The invaginated axon terminal of neuron to muscle fiber is called

a) Synaptic cleft
b) Synaptic gutter or synaptic trough
c) Synaptic space
d) None

64. An autoimmune disease where patient develops immunity against their own Ach-activated ion channels is

a) Paralysis
b) Myasthenia gravis
c) Turner syndrome
d) Gigantism

65. Actin filament is a complex protein and composed of

a) Actin
b) Tropomyosin
c) Troponin
d) All

66. Troponin I which has affinity for

a) Actin
b) Tropomyosin
c) Calcium
d) Troponin

67. Troponin T which has affinity for

a) Actin
b) Tropomyosin
c) Calcium
d) Troponin

68. Troponin C which has affinity for

a) Actin
b) Tropomyosin
c) Calcium
d) Troponin

69. Entire complex structure formed by branches of nerve fiber at its end that invaginate into muscle fiber is called

a) Synaptic space
b) Synaptic trough
c) Motor end plate
d) Synaptic gutter

70. Each myosine filament is composed of

a) One heavy chains and four light chains
b) Two heavy chains and four light chains
c) Two heavy chains and two light chains
d) Four heavy chains and four light chains

71. Length of myosin filament is of

a) 1 μm b) 1.2 μm
c) 1.6 μm d) 2.5 μm

72. Length of actin filament is of

a) 1 μm b) 1.2 μm
c) 1.6 μm d) 2.5 μm

73. Actin filament iscomposed of

a) 3 protein components b) 4 protein components
c) 5 protein components d) 6 protein components

74. Protein components of actin filament is as actin, tropomyosin and troponin

a) Actin, myosin and troponin
b) Myosine, tropomyosin and troponin
c) Actin, tropomyosin and calcium
d) Actin, tropomyosin and troponin

75. Normally in Na-K pump

a) 1 Na+ ions move to outside for each 1 K+ ions inside
b) 3 Na+ ions move to outside for each 2 K+ ions inside
c) 2 Na+ ions move to outside for each 3 K+ ions inside
d) 3 Na+ ions move to inside for each 2 K+ ions outside

76. Na-K pump is an electrogenic pump as

a) More positive charges are pumped to inside than outside
b) More negative charges are pumped to the outside than inside
c) More positive charges are pumped to the outside than inside
d) Both positive and negative charges are pumped to the outside than inside

77. Concentration gradient for Na+ ion across the resting membrane is

a) Outside-142 mEq/L, Inside–14 mEq/L
b) Outside-14 mEq/L, Inside–142 mEq/L
c) Outside-140 mEq/L, Inside–14 mEq/L
d) Outside-4 mEq/L, Inside–140 mEq/L

78. Concentration gradient for K+ ion across the resting membrane is

a) Outside-142mEq/L, Inside–14 mEq/L
b) Outside-4 mEq/L, Inside–140 mEq/L
c) Outside-14mEq/L, Inside–140 mEq/L
d) Outside-140mEq/L, Inside–4 mEq/L

79. K+ ion diffusion how much times more permeable than Na+

a) 20 times b) 40 tomes
c) 80times d) 100times

80. Recording of membrane potential and action potential is done by

a) Cathode ray oscilloscope b) Stetoscope
c) X-ray d) Sphigmomanometer

81. What is the major sources of energy for muscle contraction

a) Glycogen b) Oxidative metabolism
c) Phosphocreatine d) None

82. Muscle which deficient of myoglobin is called

a) Red muscle b) White muscle
c) Brown muscle d) All

83. Energy source of slow type fiber is

a) Oxidative or aerobic
b) Glycolytic or anaerobic
c) Both
d) Neither oxidative nor glycolytic

84. Energy source of fast type fiber is

a) Oxidative or aerobic b) Glycolytic or anaerobic
c) Both d) Neither oxidative nor glycolytic

85. Which type of skeletal muscle fiber contains large number of mitochondria

a) Slow type fiber
b) Fast type fiber
c) Both a & b contain equal number of mitochondria
d) None

86. Which fibers contain large amount of myoglobin

a) Slow type fiber
b) Fast type fiber
c) Both a & b contain equal number of myoglobin
d) None

87. Fiber having great strength of contraction

a) Slow type fiber
b) Fast type fiber
c) Both a & b have equal strength of contraction
d) None

88. Support of body weight against gravity is action of which muscle fiber

a) Slow type fiber
b) Fast type fiber
c) Both a & b
d) None

89. Jumping and running is action of which muscle fiber

a) Slow type fiber
b) Fast type fiber
c) Both a & b
d) None

90. When muscle does not shorten during contraction is called

a) Isomeric contraction
b) Isotonic contraction
c) Isovolumic contraction
d) Isometric contraction

91. When muscle is shorten with the constant tension, this contraction is called

a) Isomeric contraction
b) Isovolumic contraction
c) Isotonic contraction
d) Isometric contraction

92. Several hours after death all the muscles of the body goes into a state of contracture called

a) Muscle atrophy
b) Fatigue
c) Rigor mortis
d) Muscle twitch

93. When total mass of muscle decreases, it is called

a) Hypertrophy
b) Atrophy
c) Fatigue
d) Hyperplasia

94. When the number of muscle fibers increases, it is called

a) Hypertrophy
b) Atrophy
c) Fatigue
d) Hyperplasia

95. When total mass of muscle enlarge, it is called

a) Hypertrophy
b) Atrophy
c) Fatigue
d) Hyperplasia

96. Ciliary muscle of the eye is an example of which type muscle

a) Unitary Single unit smooth muscle
b) Multiunit smooth muscle
c) Skletal muscle
d) None

97. Smooth muscle does not contain

a) Actin
b) Myosine
c) Troponin
d) Tropomyosine

98. What is absent in smooth muscle

a) Sarcomere
b) Troponin
c) T-tubules
d) All

99. Actin filaments in smooth muscle is _______ than skeletal fiber

a) Longer
b) Shorter
c) Equal
d) None

100. Smooth muscle contain large amount of protein similar to troponin that binds to calcium is

a) Actin
b) Troponin
c) Calmodulin
d) Acetyl choline

101. Smooth muscle membrane has

a) More voltage gated Ca^{+2} channels than Na^+ channels
b) More voltage gated Na^+ channels than Ca^{+2} channels
c) Equal number of voltage gated Ca^{+2} channels than Na^+ channels
d) More voltage gated K^+ channels than Na^+ channels

102. Cell membranes that separate individual cardiac muscle cell from one another

a) Sarcomere
b) Myosine
c) Z disc
d) Intercalated discs

103. Main channel responsible for long action potential and plateau in cardiac muscle is

a) Fast Na^+ channel
b) Fast K^+ channel
c) Slow Ca^{+2} channel
d) None

104. A continuous contracted state developed in muscle due to prolonged and strong contraction is called

a) Hypertrophy
b) Titany
c) Atrophy
d) Fatigue

Answers

1. c	2. b	3. d	4. c	5. b	6. c	7. c	8. b	9. d	10. d
11. c	12. d	13. c	14. a	15. d	16. d	17. b	18. c	19. b	20. c
21. b	22. c	23. b	24. a	25. a	26. a	27. c	28. a	29. b	30. b
31. c	32. b	33. d	34. c	35. a	36. c	37. d	38. d	39. b	40. d
41. a	42. d	43. c	44. a	45. c	46. b	47. c	48. b	49. a	50. b
51. a	52. b	53. c	54. d	55. a	56. b	57. d	58. b	59. a	60. b
61. b	62. a	63. b	64. b	65. d	66. a	67. b	68. c	69. c	70. b
71. c	72. a	73. a	74. d	75. b	76. c	77. a	78. b	79. d	80. a
81. c	82. b	83. a	84. b	85. a	86. a	87. b	88. a	89. b	90.d
91. c	92. c	93. b	94. d	95. a	96. b	97. c	98. d	99. a	100. c
101. a	102. d	103. c	104. b						

❑❑❑

CHAPTER-10

Growth Physiology

Growth is defined as relatively irreversible time changes in magnitude of measured dimensions or functions. It can also be defined as the co-ordinated expression of incremental and developmental factors and functions. Body cell can be divided in terms of growth in to **renewing, expanding** and **static population**. **Prenatal growth** refers to series of differential process that transform a zygote to animal. Growth after birth is called **postnatal growth**. Prenatal growth is influenced by several factors such as heredity, size and age of dam, parity, nutrition of mother, litter size, placenta size and ambient temperature where as postnatal growth is influenced by factors like plane of nutrition, sex, heredity, hormones etc. Shape of all growth curve whether of individual or population, except man is **sigmoid**. Growth curve consists 3 phases as self accelerating phase, Point of inflection and self inhibiting phase. Point of inflection is called **point of geometric and physiologic age equivalence**. **Carbohydrate** is the principal source of energy and is usually the first limiting nutrients for the fetus. Cell division may be limited in the fetus by specific dietary deficiencies but cells may continue normally. Plane of nutrition, sex, heredity, Hormones, vitamins etc affect postnatal growth. Substances that has substantial and direct effect on growth may be classified as **growth regulators**. These growth regulators include Tissue specific growth factors, Certain hormones and Feed additives and natural occuring growth factors

Short Questions and Answers

1. **What is growth?**

Ans. Growth has been defined in many ways by different scientists. It is the co-ordinated expression of incremental and developmental factors and functions (**Hammett).** Growth is also defined as relatively irreversible time changes in magnitude of measured dimensions or functions (**Broody, 1945**). This definition of growth covers growth in size as well as weight. i.e Growth may be subdivided in to **hyperplasia** (cell multiplication), **hypertrophy** (increase in size) and **accretion** (increase in amount of non living structural matter). Growth may also defined as correlated increase in mass of the body in definite interval of time in a way characteristic of species (**Schloss, 1911**).

2. What is prenatal growth?

Ans. Prenatal growth refers to series of differential process that transform a zygote to animal. This series of process include cleavege and differentiation, organogenesis (organ formation), differential growth, hormonal regulation.

3. What is absolute growth?

Ans. It is the change in volume, crown-rump length or weight of fetus per unit of time.

4. What is relative growth?

Ans. It is absolute growth per initial dimension. Absolute growth of fetus increases exponentially with age until birth but relative growth of fetus increases during early pregnancy but then declines about midway through the gestation period.

5. What is specific growth?

Ans. In the curve of specific growth the logarithm of size is plotted against age.

6. What are the factors affect prenatal growth?

Ans. Prenatal growth is influenced by several factors such as heredity, size and age of dam, parity, nutrition of mother, litter size, placenta size and ambient temperature.

7. What are the characteristics of prenatal growth?

Ans. i) Faster prenatal growth is directly related to large maternal size

ii) Maternal contribution to variability in fetal size is greater than paternal contribution

iii) Male lambs grow larger before birth than female

iv) Poor maternal nutrition increases neonatal mortality.

v) Increase in litter size reduces rate of prenatal growth

vi) Increasing the caloric intake of the mother does not cause significant increase in fetal weight.

vii) High ambient temperature during pregnancy affects fetal size.

8. What is growth curve?

Ans. Shape of all growth curve whether of individual or population, except man is **sigmoid**. In most of the animal puberty occurs after about 30% of mature weight where as in man it is around 60-70% of mature weight. This curve consists of 3 phases **self accelerating phase, point of inflection** and **self inhibiting phase.** Shape of this growth curve is determined by two opposite forces as **growth accelerating force** that acts for self accelerating phase and **growth retarding force** that acts for self inhibiting phase.

9. What is point of inflection?

Ans. It represents the position at which the increase in growth velocity ceases but the decrease in velocity has not yet begin. Therefore inflection represents the position at which gains are most rapid and perhaps the most economical. At this point of inflection the rate of growth is same in all animal population (Numerical value of this acceleration at this time is zero). It is also called the **point of geometric and physiologic age equivalence**. Point of inflection indicates 1) Time of maximum velocity of growth 2) Age of puberty 3) Lowest specific mortality, the beginning of the period of increasing specific mortality 4) Point of geometric and physiologic age equivalence. This point of inflection is around 14yr of age in man, 5 months in cattle and 2 months for cattle.

10. What is effect of nutrition on growth?

Ans. Nutrition refers to degradation, absorption and metabolism of the food stuffs necessary for survival, growth, production and reproduction. The bioenergetics of an animal is influenced by factors as appetite and satiety which are integrative activity of central nervous system. Restriction of calorie intake greatly hampers intracellular DNA synthesis although cells continue to increase in size. On the other hand if dietary protein is restricted but caloric intake is normal cell size will be reduced but DNA accumulation continues. So both protein and caloric intake are important. Vitamins and minerals are essential for normal growth and morphogenesis. Severe deficiency or excess may cause striking change in metabolism and development of an animal. Example: Iodine deficiency inhibit normal brain development. So nutritional requirement have been estimated for several species at different ages and level of production by different experimental techniques (US national research council). **Carbohydrate** is the principal source of energy and is usually the first limiting nutrients for the fetus.

11. What is postnatal growth?

Ans. Growth after birth usually begins slowly, then goes through a rapid period and then slows down again or even may stop. **Biological definition** of growth include reproduction, increase in dimension, gain in weight, gain in organic mass, cell multiplication (mitosis), protein synthesis/metabolism etc. Growth in biological sence is connected with metabolism and organization of living system.

12. What are the factors affect postnatal growth?

Ans. The factors are plane of nutrition, sex and heredity, hormones, vitamins, antibiotics etc.

13. Growth regulators

Ans. Substance that has substantial and direct effect on growth may be classified as growth regulators. The growth regulators include

i) Tissue specific growth factors Ex. epidermal growth factor (EGF), insulin like growth factor (IGF), platelet derived growth factor (PDGF), nerve growth factor (NGF), erythropoietin, promine, retine and tissue specific chalones.

ii) Certain hormones Ex. Growth hormone, thyroid hormone, corticosteroid, androgens, estrogen

iii) Feed additives and natural occuring growth factors Ex. Synthetic hormone like compound diethyl stilbosterole (DES), synthetic estrogen, natural occuring growth factors, antibiotics, anthelmintics, tranquilizers.

Choose the Best Answer

1. Growth is defined as

a) Co-ordinated expression of incremental and developmental factors and functions

b) Relatively irreversible time changes in magnitude of measured dimensions or functions

c) Correlated increase in mass of the body in definite interval of time

d) All are correct

2. In renewing type growth tissue cells are

a) Continually lost and replaced

b) Abruptly lost and replaced

c) Neither replaced nor lost

d) All are true

3. In expanding system of growth

a) Cell division continues till death

b) Cell division continues until adult size of an organ is reached

c) Cell division does not continue

d) All are true

4. Static tissues are expanding system in which cell division is

a) Restricted to the adult stages of development

b) Cell division continues until adult size of an organ is reached

c) Restricted to the early stages of development although cellular hypertrophy occur later

d) All are true

5. Growth that refers to series of differential process that transform a zygote to animal is

a) Relative growth b) Absolute growth

c) Pre natal growth d) Post natal growth

6. Birth weight of fetus is approximately how much percentage of total weight of conceptus

a) 20% b) 40%
c) 60% d) 80%

7. Fetal membranes (Amnion, Chorioallantois, Chorionic villi) is approximately how much percentage of total weight of conceptus

a) 20% b) 40%
c) 60% d) 80%

8. Cellular division without an increase in volume is called

a) Zygote b) Cleavage
c) Morula d) Blastocyst

9. Process of establishment of organ rudiments through the interaction of germ layers is

a) Histogenesis b) Differentiation
c) Organogenesis d) All

10. Nervous system, mammary gland, hairs and hoofs are develops from

a) Mesoderm b) Endoderm
c) Ectoderm d) All

11. Interlining of the gut, its gland and bladder are develops from

a) Mesoderm b) Endoderm
c) Ectoderm d) All

12. Muscles, bones, connective tissue and vascular system are develops from

a) Ectoderm b) Endoderm
c) Mesoderm d) All

13. Cellular differentiation in which fetal tissue develop their definite characteristics are known as

a) Histogenesis b) Differentiation
c) Organogenesis d) All

14. Change in volume or weight of fetus per unit of time is called

a) Absolute growth
b) Relative growth
c) Specific growth
d) All

15. Absolute growth per initial dimension is called

a) Absolute growth
b) Relative growth
c) Specific growth
d) All

16. Faster prenatal growth is directly related to

a) Longer maternal size
b) Shorter maternal size
c) No maternal size
d) Maternal age

17. Maternal contribution to variability in fetal size is ________ than paternal contribution

a) Lesser
b) Equal
c) Greater
d) Paternal contribution is nil

18. Increase in litter size ________ rate of prenatal growth

a) Increase
b) Decrease
c) Does not affect
d) None

19. Position in the growth curve at which the increase in growth velocity ceases but the decrease in velocity has not yet begin is

a) Self Accelerating phase
b) Point of inflection
c) Self Inhibiting phase
d) None

20. Point of inflection indicates

a) Time of maximum velocity of growth
b) Point of geometric and physiologic age equivalence
c) Age of puberty
d) All

21. Metabolic rate (R) (kcal/day) is directly related to body weight (W) which is expressed by a formula as

a) $R=75W^{0.70}$
b) $R=75W^{0.95}$
c) $R=80W^{0.75}$
d) $R=70W^{0.75}$

22. Which is the principal source of energy as well as the first limiting nutrients for the fetus

a) Carbohydrate b) Protein
c) Fat d) Vitamins

23. Annual progress of a trait is calculated by a mathematical formula as

a) Annual progress of a trait = Heritability X Generation interval / Selection differential
b) Annual progress of a trait = Generation interval X Selection differential/ Heritability
c) Annual progress of a trait = Heritability - Selection differential/ Generation interval
d) Annual progress of a trait = Heritability X Selection differential/ Generation interval

24. Naturally occurring substance which is capable of stimulating cellular growth, proliferation and cellular differentiation is

a) Hormones b) Vitamins
c) Growth factor d) All

25. Growth factor that plays important role in development and life of sympathetic nerve cell is

a) Epidermal growth factor
b) Insulin like growth factor
c) Fibroblast growth factor
d) Nerve growth factor

26. Growth factor that plays significant role in blood vessel formation (angiogenesis) is

a) Epidermal growth factor
b) Insulin like growth factor
c) Platelet derived growth factor
d) Fibroblast growth factor

27. Hormonal substance circulating in blood secreted by kidney in response to hypoxia and stimulate the formation of RBC is

a) Erythropoietin b) Promine
c) Retine d) All

28. Substance that selectively inhibit mitotic activity of specific tissue is called

a) Promine
b) Retine
c) Chalones
d) Erythropoietin

29. Shape of growth curve is

a) Parabolic
b) Sigmoid
c) Hyperparabolic
d) Elliptical

30. Growth of organism reaches to steady state when anabolism and catabolism process are

a) Equal
b) Unequal
c) Zero
d) High

31. Diethyl Stilbosterole and Melengesterol acetate are

a) Synthetic progesterone
b) Synthetic estrogen
c) Synthetic testosterone
d) All

32. Growth is the most rapid in

a) Puberty
b) Childhood
c) Infancy
d) Adulthood

33. Hormone that stimulates puberty is

a) GnRH
b) LH
c) FSH
d) TSH

34. Compared to female's early growth spurt, growth is __________ and __________ in male

a) Quicker, lasts longer
b) Accelerates more slowly, lasts longer
c) Slower, shorter
d) None of the above

35. Humans are one of the _________ developing species in the animal kingdom

a) Slowest
b) Quickest
c) Average
d) None of the above

36. Expanding system of growth in which cell division is restricted to the early stage of development though cellular hypertrophy may occur later

a) Renewing
b) Expanding
c) Static tissue
d) All

Answers

1. d	2. a	3. b	4. c	5. c	6. c	7. b	8. b	9. c	10. c
11. b	12. c	13. a	14. a	15. b	16. a	17. c	18. b	19. b	20. d
21. d	22. a	23. d	24. c	25. d	26. c	27. a	28. c	29. b	30. a
31. b	32. c	33. a	34. b	35. a	36. c				

❑❑❑

CHAPTER-11

Climatology

The concept of animal adaptation refers to genetic and physiological changes takes place in an animal in response to internal and external stimuli. **Climate** is the long term (around 30 years) average condition of the meteorological variables in a given region. Meteorological variables are air temperature, humidity, air movement, radiation, barometric pressure, precipitation, rain fall, wind etc. **Weather** is the short term day to day fluctuation of the meteorological variables. Animal exchange energy/heat with its environment through radiation, convection, conduction, evaporation and metabolism. So in order for an animal to survive to a given environment over a long period of time the energy gain must be equal to energy lost. The heat loss by animal to the environment is by different means such as i) conduction ii) convection iii) radiation and iv) evaporation. The first three way of heat loss is called **sensible heat loss** where as fourth way of heat loss is called **insensible heat loss**. Animals growth and productivity is directly and indirectly affected by climatic environment. Environmental temperature is the most important climatic component affect prenatal growth. On basis of temperature regulation of body the members of animal kingdom is divided into two groups as **Homeotherm**/Endotherm/Warm blooded and **Poikilotherm**/Ectotherm/Cold blooded. **Homeotherms** are animal whose body temperature never change with the temperature of environment. They have ability to control their body temperature within narrow range in an environment. They include mammals and birds. These homeotherms are also called as **warm blooded** animals and **temperature regulators.** **Poikilotherms** are animals whose body temperature varies with the temperature of environment. They can counter act cold and heat by behavioral means but they lack almost completely physiological control of body temperature. They include reptiles and snakes. These poikilotherms are also called as **cold blooded** animals and **temperature confirmers**. The maintenance of homeothermy depends on a dynamic equilibrium between heat production and heat loss. The animal can defend itself against cold by conserving heat through insulation, by producing more heat or by a combination of both. Adaptation to cold however may involve an increase in heat production by different means. Animal can defend against heat by different means like Behavioral means, By reducing body insulation, Increasing evaporation from skin, Lowering heat production, Increasing heat reflectance of hair coat to solar radiation. There are three basic components of temperature regulating system in body as sensor, thermostatic control unit and thermoregulating effectors (Heat loss and Heat produce). So the body system functions as a thermostat with a **set point** (desired core temperature).

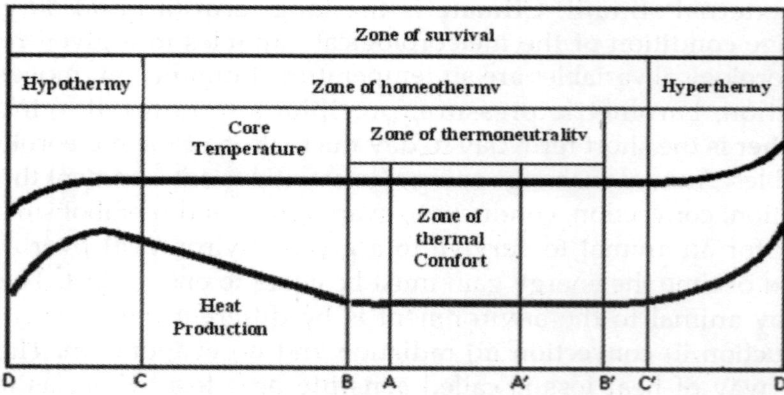

Zones of environment

Short Questions and Answers

1. **What is climate?**

Ans. **Climate** is the long term (around 30 years) average condition of the meteorological variables in a given region. Meteorological variables are air temperature, humidity, air movement, radiation, barometric pressure, precipitation, rain fall, wind etc. Climate is of two types as macroclimate and microclimate. **Macroclimate** is the general large scale climatic condition of an open atmosphere in a large area or country. **Microclimate** is the climatic condition directly surrounding the animal.

2. What is weather?

Ans. It is the short term day to day fluctuation of the meteorological variables or instantaneous value of these meteorological variables. Climate of a region has a profound influence on the animals living there. Animals life is geared to the seasonal rhythm of plant growth and decline. Climate directly affects directly on the growth of animal through its control over their heat exchange through neuroendocrine and behavioral means.

3. Related definition of Climatology?

Ans. **Adaptation (Biological):** It refers to morphological, anatomical, Physiological, biochemical and behavioral characteristics of animal which promotes welfare and favor survival in a specific environment.

Adaptation (Genetic): It refers to heritable animal characteristics which favor survival of a population in a particular environment. This may involve evolutionary changes over many generations (selection by nature) or acquiring specific genetic properties (selection by man).

Adaptation (Physiological): It is the capacity and process of adjustment of animal to itself, to other living materials and to its external physical environment.

Acclimatization: It refers to a long term adaptive physiological adjustment which results in an increased tolerance to continuous and repeated exposure to complex climatic stressors/variables (normally produced in field condition).

Acclimation: It refers to adaptive changes in response to a single climatic variable (normally produced in climatic chamber).

Habituation (General): It is a gradual quantitative change of response which may lead to a loss of response as a result of repeated stimulus.

Habituation (Specific): It is the gradual reduction in sensation associated with a given repeated stimulus specific to the part of body which has been repeatedly stimulated

Learning: It is the acquisition of a new response or qualitative change of an existing response or an inhibition or facilitation of an existing response by a new stimulus.

Conditioning: It is the transfer of an existing response to a new stimulus.

Biological rhythm: Many biological activities of animals are repeated after a particular time interval in a cyclic manner. This cyclic manner is called as biological rhythm.The repeatatin of such activities within 24 hour period of the day is called as **circadian rhythm** or **diurnal rhythm**.

Ultradian and infradian: There are variety of other rhythms which are shorter and longer than circadian rhythm. Shorter rhythms are called **ultradian** and longer rhythms are called **infradian**. Example of ultradian is release of luteinizing hormone and example of infradian is sexual cycle.e during winter.

Estivation: It is a condition of sleep like inactivity during summer which is analogous to hibernation in winter to survive on low energy balance and to conserve body water.

Hibernation: It is the state of winter inactivity in homeothermic animals during which there is reduction in locomotion, body temetrature, BMR, heart rate and respiration rate duinng winter.

Hemostasis: Hemostasis is a reaction of the animal to any non specific environment involving pituitary-thyroid- adrenal axis which tries to place the body in a physiological state.

Hemothermism: It is a condition of maintaining the body temperature to a particular point irrespective of the change in environmental temperature. The animals of this category are called homeotherms or warm blooded animals.

Poikilotherms: It is a state of changing the body temperature with change in environmental temperature. The animals of this category are called poikilotherms or cold blooded animals.

4. What are ecological rules regarding morphological adaptation?

Ans. There are four ecological rules regarding morphological adaptation. They are as such

Bergmann's rule: The smaller size breeds of a given species are found in the warmer parts of the ecological range. The larger size breeds are in the cooler area.

Allen's rule: The protruding body organs like extrimities, tails, ears are relatively shorter in the cooler parts of the ecological range than in the warmer areas.

Wilson's rule: Insulation cover based on the length of the hair and thickness of adipose tissue is related to climate.

Golger's rule: Mammalian and avian breeds which inhabit in warm and humid regions have more melanin pigmentation than those of the same species in the cooler and drier region.

5. **What are the means of heat loss by animal to the environment?**

Ans. The heat loss by animal to the environment is by different means such as i) conduction ii) convection iii) radiation and iv) evaporation. The first three way of heat loss is called **sensible heat loss** where as fourth way of heat loss is called **insensible heat loss**. Heat transfer by radiation, convection and conduction can operate in opposite direction i.e from environment to the body but heat transfer by evaporation is only away from body.

i) **Conduction**

It is the transfer of heat through a medium without transfer of materials.

ii) **Convection**

It refers to the transfer of heat by streams of molecules from warm object to a less warm object.

iii) **Radiation**

The flow of heat by radiation does not depend upon the temperature or movement of the ambient air but only on the temperature and nature of the surface of the radiating body.

iv) **Evaporation**

Here humidity plays role. The vapour pressure of water at the skin, the surrounding air, air velocity also affects evaporation. This evaporation is by water from skin and respiratory passage. The evaporation of 1 kg of water from body requires about 575 kcal depending upon the temperature of the evaporating surface, temperature and humidity of air. In otherwise evaporation decreases with increasing air humidity.

6. What are the factors affect heat production?

Ans. Factors affecting heat production are

i) **Ingestion of food:** Ingestion of food leads to an increase in heat production. The calori genetic effect of the food varies with the class of nutrients ingested. It is highest in protein. The faster turnover of food in the growing as compared with the adult animal is associated with an increased heat production.

ii) **Microorganism in rumen:** In ruminants microorganisms constitutes an extra source of heat contributing upto 10% of animals basal heat production.

iii) **Muscular activity:** It also increases heat production. In cattle and sheer heat production is about 10% greater during standing than lying.

iv) **Pregnancy:** Pregnancy also increases heat production. Metabolism of fetus together with acceleration of various body process of mother increases heat production in pregnant animal.

v) **Lactation:** Lactation leads to increase in heat production.

7. What is the effect of climate on growth and production?

Ans. Animals growth and productivity is directly and indirectly affected by climatic environment. Indirectly temperature, humidity, air movement, solar radiation, rain fall or barometric pressure affect the plane of nutrition of animal through the amount of crops and pastures. A direct environmental consequences is the stimulation of neuroendocrine system resulting in the loss or conservation of heat to maintain body temperature within he narrow optimal range of biological activity. Growth is a complex set of metabolic events which are environmentally or genetically controlled. Among the climatic condition that impose stress on the rate of prenatal, preweaning and postweaning growth are temperature, humidity, air movement and radiation. The climatic conditions also affects the amount of food and water intake, the availability of potential energy in the ingested forage, heat production system, the net energy available for productivity and the body composition of growing animals.

8. What is the effect of climate on milk yield and milk composition?

Ans. Milk biosynthesis depends on mammary gland receiving a continuous supply of various metabolites and hormone from blood. The milk yield of all mammalian species undergoes seasonal variations. In cattle the yield is relatively unaffected within range of temperature of 5-21°C. At the temperature less than 5°C as well as from 21-27°C the yield decreases slowly where as above 27°C the decline is much more marked. This decline is more marked in high humid in comparison to low humid condition. It has been estimated that milk production decreases approximately 1kg for each degree rise in rectal temperature. The optimal environmental temperature for lactation is dependent on species, breed and degree of tolerance o heat and cold. There is also breed difference in the maximal and minimal critical temperature beyond which productivity decreases rapidly. Ex. In Holstein cow milk yield declines at 21°C, in brown swiss and jersey breed milk yield declines at 24-27°C and in Brahma breed this decline is seen at 32°C. The minimal critical temperature for jersey breed is at 2°C where as Holstein are not greatly affected even a -13°C. However at 35°C and relative humidity of 25% there is drop in feed consumption and milk production. Some of the milk constituents like NPN of cattle exposed to high environmental temperature increases but constituents like fat, total solids, solid not fat, lactose, short chain fatty acids, calcium, potassium decreases but there is no change in sodium concentration in milk. Low ambient temperature cause increase in butter fat percentage. Total solids, total nitrogen and solid not fat are also greater at temperature below freezing than at 10°C.

9. What is the effect of climate on wool growth?

Ans. The response of wool growth to environment varies according to the breed of sheep, physical condition of the animals, plane of nutrition, sex, seasonal and diurnal variation, environmental temperature and photo period. Maximum growth of wool occurs in summer and minimal growth occurs in winter, it implies winter prevents wool growth. Sheep given artificial heating for period of three months during winter results an increase in wool growth. Both thyroid and adrenal gland activity affects wool growth. Adrenal cortical hormone prevents wool growth. Photoperiod also affects wool growth i.e shorter day length decreases wool growth independent upon temperature changes.

10. What is the effect of temperature on male reproduction?

Ans. The scrotum behaves like a thermostat holding the testes close to the body when the air temperature is below 6°C. The testes drops to maximum distance from the body when the air temperature is above 24°C. In all domestic animals spermatogenesis is depressed at body temperature. The quantity and quality of semen varies with the season of the year. In summer semen characteristics are inferior or in many cases semen is not ejaculated. Summer sterility in ram is common a latitude of 35° or more. Horse semen is produced throughout the year but the gelatinous material which constitutes half of the ejaculate is highest during spring and summer season.

11. What is the effect of photoperiod on male reproduction?

Ans. The generation time of primary spermatocytes and the time for subsequent maturation are relatively unaffected by the photoperiod. The maintenance of constant photoperiod for 35-40 days results a decline in spermatogenesis.

12. What is the effect of climate on female reproduction?

Ans. **Puberty:** The season of birth affects he age at which puberty will occur mainly in animals. Body weight of the ewe at her first estrus and conception are minimal if she was born in the spring and maximal if born in summer. Cattle reach puberty at an average of 13 months t 27°C and 10 months at 10°C. Sexual activity in mammal is primarily controlled by dark-light ratio.

Estrus cycle and ovulation: Seasonal variations in length of estrus cycle and duration of estrus are not marked in species with short cycle or living near equator. The estrus cycle in horse is prolonged during spring and gradually shorter there after. High temperature don't affect the length of estrus cycle in sheep and swine. Heat stress in cattle cause shortening of estrus duration.

Fertilization and conception: Thermal stress causes morphological abnormalities of eggs like shrinkage of cytoplasm, rupture vielline membrane, ruptured zona pellucid etc. In sheep fertilization rate is reduced if exposed to 32°C. The conception rate in cattle is greater in spring than summer. Possibly the increasing day length and moderate temperature of spring are optimal condition for conception. In tropic and sub tropics conception rate of water buffalo is greatly influenced by the season of the year which is being lowest during summer.

Gestation and fetal development: Extreme high temperature, lower fertility, decrease litter size, increase abortion and increase fetal resorption. Among the domestic animals horse have wide seasonal variation in gestation. It is lowest for mares foaling in spring or summer.

Neonatal survive: Upon birth the neonates must make thermoregulatory adjustment to fluctuating environmental condition. The efficiency of such adjustment depends primarily on the degree of physiological immaturity of the species at birth. Swine and sheeps are susceptible to low temperature. Lambs at age of 2-7 days cann't survive longer than two hours at 38°C or more than three hours of solar radiation exposure.

13. What is the effect of climate on egg production in birds?

Ans. The environment markedly affects age and weight of birds at sexual maturity, total number of eggs laid per clutch per season and per year and egg weight also. An increase in day length advanced the onset of sexual maturity. Spring is the sexual season for most birds in the temperate zones. In domestic fowls under natural environments the intensity of egg production is associated more or less with long days of the year. Continuous light for 24 hours a day stimulates winter egg production. Within the range of 9-29°C egg production in domestic fowls is not reduced. Thermal stress especially sharp change in temperature adversely affects both egg weight and shell quality. A 24 hour exposure to 38°C resulted a sudden temporary drop in egg production of some strains but not others. Temperature above 32°C shell thickness of egg decreases.

14. What is thermal balance?

Ans. The maintenance of homeothermy depends on a dynamic equilibrium between heat production and heat loss. In simplest form thermal balance is expressed as **Heat production= Heat loss ± Heat storage.** The storage capacity per unit surface area is greater in large animals than in small animals. Maintenance of a steady thermal state in cold and hot environments has been expressed by Burton and Edholm as

$$M = \frac{Tc - Ta}{It + Icl + Ia} + E$$

Here M= Metabolic rate

Tc = Temperature of body core

Ta = Temperature of environment

It = Insulation of tissue

Icl = Insulation of clothing or hair coat

Ia = Insulation of air

E = Evaporation

15. How animal defence against heat?

Ans. Heat refers to meteorological elements which either oppose the flow of excess heat from the animal to environment or which promote transfer of thermal energy from environment to animal. The most important ones are environmental temperature, air humidity and solar radiation. Air movement has a heating effect only when air temperature is above body surface temperature which occurs rarely.The animal can defend against heat by different means like i) Behavioral means ii) By reducing body insulation iii) Increasing evaporation from skin iv) Lowering heat production v) Increasing heat reflectance of hair coat to solar radiation.

16. How body temperature is regulated?

Ans. There are three basic components of temperature regulating system as sensor, thermostatic control unit and thermoregulating effectors (Heat loss and Heat produce). So the body system functions as a thermostat with a **set point** (desired core temperature). The thermoregulatory control centre lies in the hypothalamus. The anterior region of hypothalamus chiefly concern with prevention of over cooling. It mainly associated with heat loss from body and certain warm receptors. Where as posterior part of hypothalamus is associated with heat production by body and certain cold receptors. In anterior hypothalamus heat loss is by peripheral vasodilation, sweating and panting. In posterior hypothalamus heat production is by shivering and non shivering means. Shivering method is by involuntary contraction of skeletal muscle and oxygen consumption. Non-shivering means is by behavioral means and by hormonal action. Hormones like Thyroid, epinephrine and nor epinephrine plays role here. Increase secretion of these hormones occurs in mammals during cold stress.

17. Which is more stressful fever or hyperthermia?

Ans. There is evidence that the temperature which the body tries to maintain is called set point which is not rigidly fixed but it changes within limit. In **fever** the set point is raised due to pyrogens. The thermoregulatory mechanism in fever remains fully intact but they operate at a higher level of core temperature. So the thermoregulatory mechanism is little affected in fever. But in **hyperthermia** the thermoregulatory mechanism is fully activated. Therefore **hyperthermia is more stressful than fever**.

18. What are zones of environmental temperature?

Ans. The range of environmental temperature within which body temperature is maintained constant with a minimal effort from thermoregulatory mechanism and within which the sensation of heat or cold is absent. In human this range is called as **comfort zone**. In this zone blood vessels of the skin over the whole body are neither all vasodilated nor all vasoconstricted. Here evaporation of moisture is minimal. Piloerection and behavioral responses to heat and cold are absent. Moving out of zone of thermal comfort towards heat and cold, animal activates its defence mechanism. When environmental temperature falls below thermal comfort general vasoconstriction and piloerection takes place which bring about some increase in heat conservation. With the temperature falling further beginning at some point called **lower critical temperature** where rate of heat production rises. At still lower temperature at some point the extra heat production is insufficient to balance heat loss from the animal and the body temperature begins to fall. So heat production after reaching a peak declines sharply thereby accelerating the cooling process. Eventually at some point animal dies from cold. Similarly when environmental temperature rises above thermal comfort physical defence mechanism against over heating comes to operation by vasodilation, sweating, panting etc. When the temperature rises further a point called **upper critical temperature where** sweating and panting becomes intensified and there is compensatory decrease in heat production. If still the temperature rises sweating, panting or both are further increased but cooling by this is insufficient to maintain homeothermy of body. So the body temperature begins to rise. This is inturn increases metabolic rate. When further increases temperature there is death of animal.

19. How bird regulate body temperature?

Ans. The internal temperature of birds is higher than that of mammals. Deep body temperature of common d0omestic species like pigeon, ducks, geese, turkey and chicken range from 41.2°C to 42.2°C. There are several inherent factors which influence deep body temperature. Newly hatched chicks have body temperature approximately 2.5°C below those of adult birds. This increase temperature is related to feather covers and increased metabolic activity associated with growth. Body temperature also varies with size, sex and breed. Generally males have high temperature than female. White leghorn have high temperature than new Hampshire. Increased physical activity, caloric intake and environmental temperature tends to increase body temperature. To maintain homeothermy several anatomical systems interact including the outer integument, respiratory system, cardio vascular system and nervous system.

20. What are different instruments/equipments used to record climatic variables?

Ans. Various climatic variables include air temperature, relative air humidity, air movement, barometric pressure and amount of solar radiation. To study on different climatic variables following instruments are used

i) **Stevenson screen:** It is a **wooden rectangular box** of dimensions 2′ x 2.5′ x 2.75′ feet having louvered walls to permit free movement of air and to protect the instruments placed inside from sunshine, rain and snow. It has the double roof, the lower roof being horizontal and the upper roof is inclined backward. Between the two roofs the air can move freely. The upper part of roof prevents radiations. Circulation of air between the two roofs prevents the lower roof from becoming hot. The box is placed at about 4 feet height from the leveled ground. The bottom prevents the radiations from the earth reaching the instruments. On the stand inside minimum, maximum, dry and wet bulb thermometers, thermograph and hygrograph are placed.

ii) **Vernon globe thermometer:** A standard globe thermometer consists of a hollow copper sphere about 15 cm in diameter, the exterior of which is evenly painted black. It is fitted with an ordinary mercury thermometer having its bulb at the center of sphere. It is **used to record the mean radiation** of the surrounding as cal/ cm2/sec.

iii) **Kata thermometer:** It is a special type of alcohol thermometer to record cooling power of the air. It has two marks on its stem. The marks may be at the level of 95 and 100ºF or 125 and 130ºF or 145 and 150ºF. Kata is heated by immersing it in hot water until the alcohol level is above the top mark. It is then wiped dry and the time is noted for the alcohol to fall from the top to the bottom mark. Each kata thermometer is marked with a factor which when divided by the average cooling time in second gives the so called cooling power as millicalories/cm2/sec. It is **used to measure the rate of cooling** of the air in rooms or halls.

iv) **Sunshine recorder:** It is a solid spherical glass ball used to **record the duration of sunshine**. A hard paper strip graduated in hours of the day is placed at the focal length of the ball. The sunrays focusing through the ball char the strip depending on the appearance of the sunshine.

v) **Lux meter:** This instrument is used to record the light intensity of range between 1-2,00,000 Lux in a temperature range between 0-40°C and relative humidity to ≤ 80 %. A photo detector, which senses the light intensity, may be held at the desired level of ground under light source. It displays the **light intensity** in lux.

vi) **Cup anemometer:** It consists of three or four hemispherical aluminum or copper cups attached at the end of arms. The arms are connected to the vertical spindle. When it is exposed to wind, the cups move about its axis with convex surface foremost. As the cups move, vertical spindle rotates which transmits motion to the recording system. The circular scale of recording system **gives the speed of wind.**

vii) **Wind-vane:** It has a balanced lever that turns freely about a vertical axis. One end of lever is broad and bifurcated, this is known as fang. Other end is narrow and points to the direction from which the wind blows; this is known as pointer or arrowhead. Under this movable system a rigid cross arm is fixed and set to the four cardinal directions N.,E.,S. and W. Some wind-vanes are provided with eight directions. It is installed over a wooden post or fixed on the concrete platform. The distance between the pointer and ground level should be exactly 10 feet. The north indicator should be set to true North and not to the magnetic North. This instrument measures the direction of wind.

viii) **Rain gauge:** It consists of four parts. 1.Funnel 2.Receiver 3. Body 4. Measuring cylinder. This funnel is produced with a brass rim, which should be truly circular and 5" in diameter. The height of the rain gauge should be 12" above the ground level and 10" above cemented platform. The rain is collected in receiver and measured by a standard measuring cylinder (4 cm diameter) provided with the instrument (1 cm = 1 mm rain).

ix) **Evaporation pan:**

It is a large circular container having depth of 25 cm and a diameter of 120 cm. The wall and the base are made up of iron sheet. A metallic rod (19 cm long) is fixed in the center of heavy walled cylinder (10 cm inner diameter) such that the rounded tip of the rod projects out of the cylinder. At 7.00 AM the cylinder is kept in the pan up to the level of the tip of the rod of the cylinder. Pan is then covered with wire mesh so that the birds may not drink water contained in the pan. At 2.00 PM, clean water is added up to the level of the tip of the rod with the help of small metallic bucket graduated up to 20 cm. Each cm of water **added indicates 1mm of evaporation**.

Choose the Best Answer

1. **Panting is not observed in**

a) Dog b) Horse
c) Cat d) Poultry

2. **Rate of mitosis is affected by**

a) Heredity and sex b) Nutrition
c) Ambient Temperature d) All

3. **During Fear and excitement there may be**

a) Rise in heart rate and respiration rate
b) Increased release of epinephrine and ACTH
c) Rise in systolic blood pressure
d) All of above

4. Torpid sleeping state during summer refers to

a) Hibernation b) Aestivation
c) Hibituation d) None of the above

5. Adaptive changes in the response to a single climatic variable is known as

a) Adaptation b) Habituation
c) Acclimation d) Conditioning

6. In which of the following process the heat transfer from the body is in one direction

a) Radiation b) Conduction
c) Convection d) Evaporation

7. Which of the following is a non-sweating species

a) Sheep b) Goat
c) Cattle d) Pig

8. Thermo-regulatory control center lies in

a) Cerebral cortex b) Hypothalamus
c) Cerebellum d) None of these

9. The zone of thermo neutrality in most of the animal is

a) 15-28°C b) 5-15°C
c) 30-37°C d) 0-30°C

10. The instrumentused for the continuous recording of temperature is known as

a) Thermograph
b) Psychrometer
c) Dry and wet bulb thermometer
d) All

11. Wool growth is maximum in

a) Summer b) Winter
c) Spring d) All

12. Metabolic heat production is more in

a) Large animals b) Medium animals
c) Small animals d) None of the above

13. Depending up on the strategies and regulation of body temperatures the animals are classified as

a) Ruminants and non ruminants
b) Domestic and wild
c) Vertebrates and non vertebrates
d) Homeotherms and poikilotherms

14. Sweet gland is absent in

a) Dog b) Cattle
c) Horse d) Goat

15. Long term average condition of the meteorological variables in a given region is

a) Weather b) Climate
c) Microclimate d) Macroclimate

16. Large scale climatic condition of an open atmosphere in a large area or country is

a) Weather b) Climate
c) Microclimate d) Macroclimate

17. Short term day to day fluctuation of the meteorological variables is

a) Weather b) Climate
c) Microclimate d) Macroclimate

18. Climatic condition directly surrounding the animal is

a) Weather b) Climate
c) Microclimate d) Macroclimate

19. Climate types which can be found in low latitude areas are

a) Arid and Medierranean b) Tropical wet and Dry
c) Highland and Subtropicl d) Gighland and Dry

20. Rotation of the earth causes

a) Greenhouse effect b) Night and day
c) Climate changes d) Changing seasons

21. Elevation and Latitude affect

a) How rivers flow
b) Climate
c) Boundaries between different countries
d) Night and Day

22. Doldrums are

a) Areas where the tradewinds flow westward
b) Polar easterlies
c) Winds that bring wet and dry weather
d) Areas near equator with very little wind

23. Arid and Semiarid climate types are both

a) High latitude climate types
b) Classified as dry
c) Found only in North America and Africa
d) None

24. Our climate type is

a) Humid continental
b) Mediterranean
c) West coast marine
d) Humid subtropical

25. Tropical wet climate type can be described as

a) Hot all year with a wet and a dry season
b) Hot summers with cool winters
c) Varying greatly depending on elevation
d) Hot and wet all year

26. Climate type which has hot temperatures all year and has both a wet and a dry season

a) Tropical wet
b) Humid subtropical
c) Humid continental
d) Tropical wet and dry

27. Qualitative change of an existing response by a new stimulus is called

a) Conditioning
b) Habituation
c) Learning
d) None

28. When it is winter in the Northern hemisphere, in the southern hemisphere it is

a) Spring b) Summer
c) Fall d) Winter

29. Transfer of an existing response to a new stimulus

a) Conditioning b) Habituation
c) Learning d) None

30. Gradual quantitative change of response as a result of repeated stimulus is called

a) Conditioning b) Habituation
c) Learning d) None

31. All moderate or seasonal climates can be found in

a) Low latitude areas b) Middle latitude areas
c) High latitude areas d) All

32. On a climate graph, precipitation is shown by

a) A bar that comes up from the bottom of the graph
b) A line that goes across the graph
c) Both
d) None

33. On a climate graph, temperature is shown by

a) A bar that comes up from the bottom of the graph
b) A line that goes across the graph
c) Both
d) None

34. Side of the mountain facing wind receiving more rain than the other side of the mountain is

a) Typical of lands with moderate climates
b) Called as orographic effect
c) Rarely found on tropical islands
d) All are correct

35. Savanna's are tropical grasslands near the equator that

a) Have tall grasses and a few scattered trees
b) Support abundant wildlife with thick, jungle-like vegetation
c) Receive a lot of precipitation in both the winter and summer seasons
d) All are correct

36. A change of season is caused by

a) Earth's rotation b) Earth's revolution.
c) Earth's tilt. d) b &c

37. Capacity and process of adjustment of animal to itself, to other living materials and to its external physical environment is

a) Habituation b) Learning
c) Adaptation d) Conditioning

38. Transfer of heat through a medium without transfer of material is called

a) Conduction b) Convection
c) Radiation d) Evaporation

39. Sweat glands are absent in

a) Cattle b) Human
c) Horse d) Dog

40 Long term adaptive physiological adjustment to complex climatic stressors is called

a) Acclimation b) Acclimatization
c) Weather d) Climate

41. Adaptive changes in response to a single climatic variable is called

a) Acclimation b) Acclimatization
c) Weather d) Climate

42. Way of insensible heat loss is

a) Conduction b) Convection
c) Radiation d) Evaporation

43 Way of sensible heat loss is

a) Conduction b) Convection
c) Radiation d) All

44. Transfer of heat through a medium without transfer of materials is

a) Conduction b) Convection
c) Radiation d) Evaporation

45. To survive in a given environment over a long period of time the energy gain by an animal must be— — to the energy loss

a) More b) Less
c) Equal d) None

46. The seasonal changes of day length control breeding cycle of which species

a) Canine b) Ovine
c) Feline d) Caprine

47. Rate of evaporation _______ with increase in humidity

a) Decrease b) Increase
c) Not affected d) None

48. Pregnant ewes exposed to high temperature leads to which condition in lambs

a) Heat induced dwarfism b) Mental retardation
c) Growth retardation d) All

49. Climatic condition directly surrounding to animal is called

a) Climate b) Micro-climate
c) Macro-climate d) Weather

50. Loss of heat through radiation is called _______ heat loss

a) Sensible b) Insensible
c) Both a & b d) None

51. The oil producing gland present in bird is

a) Sebaceous gland b) Sweat gland
c) Preen gland d) All

52. The repetition of biological activity in every 24 hr is known as

a) Circadian rhythm b) Biological rhythm
c) Physiological rhythm d) All

53. Birth weight of fetus is approximately _______ % of total weight of conceptus

a) 20% b) 40%
c) 60% d) 80%

54. Transfer of heat by streams of molecules from warm object to a less warm object is

a) Conduction b) Convection
c) Radiation d) Evaporation

55. Humidity plays role in which type of heat loss

a) Conduction b) Convection
c) Radiation d) Evaporation

56. Evaporation of 1 kg of water from body requires about

a) 475 kcal heat b) 390 kcal heat
c) 575 kcal heat d) 515 kcal heat

57. Summer sterility is common in

a) Horse b) Dog
c) Lamb d) Sheep

58. Minimum critical temperature for Jersey cattle is

a) 2°C b) 4°C
c) 8°C d) 10°C

59. Minimum critical temperature for Holstein cattle is

a) 2°C b) 4°C
c) -8°C d) -13°C

60. Domestic animal which has widest seasonal variation is

a) Sheep b) Goat
c) Pig d) Horse

61. Posterior part of hypothalamus is associated with

a) Heat production b) Heat receiver
c) Over cooling d) Over heating

62. Stage which is affected by heat stress during pregnancy is

a) Implantation stage b) Zygotic stage
c) Blastocyst stage d) Embryonic stage

63. Smaller size breeds of a given species are found in the warmer parts of the ecological range implies which ecological rules

a) Bergmann's rule b) Allen's rule
c) Wilson's rule d) Golger's rule

64. Protruding body organs are relatively shorter in the cooler parts of the ecological range than in the warmer areas implies which ecological rules

a) Bergmann's rule b) Allen's rule
c) Wilson's rule d) Golger's rule

65. Insulation cover based on the length of the hair and thickness of adipose tissue is related to climate implies which ecological rules

a) Bergmann's rule b) Allen's rule
c) Wilson's rule d) Golger's rule

66. Mammalian and avian breeds which inhabit in warm and humid regions have more melanin pigmentation than those of the same species in the cooler and drier region implies which ecological rules

a) Bergmann's rule b) Allen's rule
c) Wilson's rule d) Golger's rule

67. Organ that has lowest oxygen consumption/ 100gm/minute

a) Skeletal Muscle b) Heart
c) Liver d) Brain

68. Organ that has highest oxygen consumption/ 100gm/minute

a) Skeletal Muscle b) Heart
c) Liver d) Brain

69. Metabolic rate is more nearly proportional to the

a) 1/2 of the body weight
b) 3/4th power of body weight
c) 2/5th power of body weight
d) None

70. Animal whose body temperature never change with the temperature of environment

a) Homeotherms b) Poikilotherm
c) Both d) None

71. Animal whose body temperature varies with the temperature of environment

a) Homeotherms b) Poikilotherm
c) Both d) None

72. Environmental temperature below which heat production begins to increase in defence against cold is termed as

a) Lower critical temperature b) Upper critical temperature
c) Critical temperature d) Neutral temperature

73. Body system functions as a thermostat with a desired core temperature called

a) Dew point b) Neutral point
c) Set point d) Core point

Answers

1. b	2. d	3. d	4. b	5. c	6. d	7. d	8. b	9. a	10. a
11. a	12. a	13. d	14. a	15 .b	16. d	17. a	18. c	19. b	20. b
21. b	22. d	23. b	24. a	25. d	26. d	27. c	28. b	29. a	30. b
31. b	32. a	33. b	34. b	35. a	36. d	37. c	38. a	39. d	40. b
41. a	42. d	43. d	44. a	45. c	46. b	47. a	48. a	49. b	50. b
51. c	52. a	53. c	54. b	55. d	56. c	57. d	58. a	59. d	60. d
61. a	62. b	63. a	64. b	65. c	66. d	67. a	68. d	69. b	70. a
71. b	72. a	73. c							

□□□

CHAPTER-12

Lactation Physiology

Mammary gland is the milk secreting structure, which includes a **teat**, a **duct system** and **lobes** (lobules) of secretory tissue drained by the duct system. Mammary glands are modified sweat (sudoriferous) glands which secretes milk (exocrine gland) and serve as accessory glands to the reproductive system. Udder is a complex organ made up of a series of systems, which includes a supportive system, secretory system composed of epithelial cells, a duct system for storage and conveyance of milk and blood, lymph and nerve systems. The udder of the cow is supported by two major groups of ligaments as **median suspensory ligaments (MSL) and lateral suspensory ligaments (LSL). Mammary gland** consists of connective tissue, ductular system and secretory tissue. The function of the connective tissue is to support the ductular and the secretory tissues. A desirable udder should contain a minimal amount of connective tissue and maximal amounts of secretory tissue. The ductular system of the mammary gland starts at the alveoli and ends at the streak canal. The secretory epithelial cells comprise about 1/2 of the total cells in the secretory tissue during lactation. Secretory tissue is arranged into **lobes** with each lobes consists of many **lobules**. Each lobule containing clusters or groups of **alveoli** (150-220 alveoli) which are surrounded by a network of blood vessels. Each alveolus has all the components required to produce and deliver milk to the duct system. The rate at which blood flow to the mammary gland is one of the key factors in determining milk synthetic rate. It takes from 400 to 500 ml of blood flowing the mammary glands to produce one ml of milk.

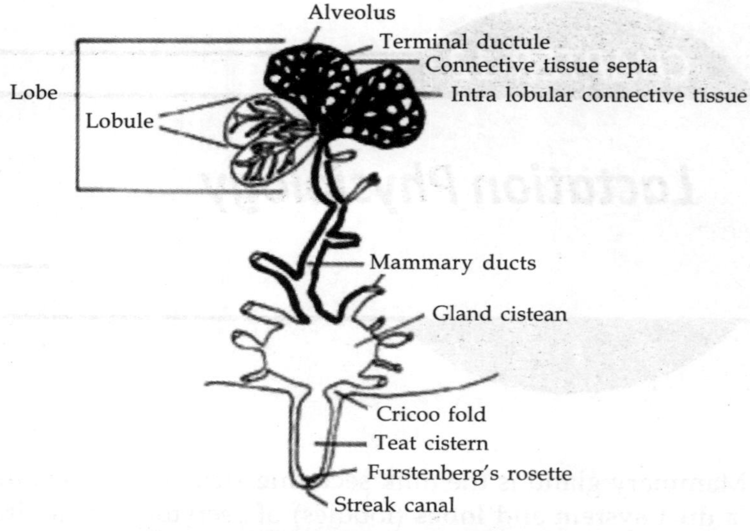

Crosssection of Mammary Gland

Ejection of milk is accomplished by contraction of the myoepithelial cells surrounding each alveolus. The ejection process results in a rapid transfer of milk from the lobulo-alveolar spaces into larger ducts. Milk ejection is a neurohormonal reflex associated with the release of **oxytocin**. Milk ejection reflex has a neural (afferent) and a hormonal (efferent) component. Milk is composed of water, carbohydrate, fat, protein, minerals and vitamins. It is important to remember that milk is secreted as a complex mixture of these components. The properties and importance of milk are greater and more complex than the sum of its components. There is a considerable variability in the number of glands and location along the midline among mammalian species. **Anterior:** Include primates, elephants, sea cows, bats and **Posterior:** Include ungulates, whales. Mammogenesis is the term use to describe the development of the mammary gland. Mammary development begins when the animal is an early fetus and proceeds beyond initiation of lactation. The major portion of mammary growth occurs during pregnancy and is controlled by hormones. Growth of the mammary gland is slow at the beginning of pregnancy but the rate of growth accelerates as the pregnancy advances. Mammogenesis during pregnancy has been shown to be exponential in cattle, goats and guinea pigs. In the mammary gland of non-pregnant females a large fatty pad exists. As pregnancy progresses the adipose cells of the pad are gradually replaced by ducts, alveoli, blood vessels and connective tissue. **Alveoli are not formed before pregnancy is established**. Both estrogen and progesterone are required for optimal mammary growth. Initiation of milk secretion is called as **Lactogenesis.** It is a series of cellular changes whereby mammary epithelial cells are converted from a non secretory state to a secretory state. This process is normally associated with the end of pregnancy and around the time of parturition. Lactogenesis is a two stage process as **stage I** (Cytologic and enzymatic differentiation of alveolar epithelial cells) and **stage II** (Copious secretion of all milk components). **Galactopoeisis** is defined as the maintenance of lactation or milk secretion once lactation has been established. The changes in mammary cell numbers (by growth or cell death) and in milk yield per cell are regulated by galactopoietic hormones and local mammary factors.

Short Questions and Answers

1. **What is mammary gland?**

Ans. Mammary gland is the milk secreting structure, which includes a **teat**, a **duct system** and **lobes** (lobules) of secretory tissue drained by the duct system. Mammary glands are modified sweat (sudoriferous) glands which secretes milk (exocrine gland) and serve as accessory glands to the reproductive system.

2. **What is supportive system of udder?**

Ans. A stronger udder supportive (suspensory) system is required to maintain proper attachments of the gland to the body. The udder of the cow is supported by two major groups of ligaments as

i) **Median Suspensory Ligaments (MSL):** The most important part of the suspensory system in cows. The MSL divide the udder into two distinct halves and provide the primary support for the udder. When the cow is viewed from behind a distinct midline groove marks the position of median suspensory ligament.

ii) **Lateral Suspensory Ligaments (LSL):** These structures contain more collagen than elastin and thus provide support but not elasticity to the udder. The LSL arise from the above and posterior to the udder and extend along both sides of the udder providing support to the interior of the udder. The LSL extend to the midline on the floor of the udder joining the MSL at the base of the udder. The skin provides the udder with protection but with little support. The udder is attached to the skin by a **fine connective tissue** and a **coarse connective tissue** attaches the forequarters to the abdominal wall.

3. What is the structure of teat?

Ans. Cows have four teats (one teat drains on gland). The skin of the teat is characterized by the absence of hair and glands (sweat or sebaceous glands). Teat size and shape is independent of the size, shape or milk production of the udder.

Teat (streak) canal: It is closed by circular sphincter muscles. The streak canal retains the milk in the udder against the pressure developed by the accumulation of milk. It is also the main barrier against infection and is lines with skinlike epidermis cells that produce a bacteriostatic secretion.

Furstenburg's rosette: Mucosal folds of the streak canal lining at the internal end of the canal. It folds over the canal opening due to pressure when the udder is full, which aids in he retention of milk. It may be a major point of entry for leukocytes leaving the teat lining and entering the into the teat cistern.

Annular (cricoid) rings: Located at the proximal end of the teat cistern, marking the boundary between the teat cistern and the gland cistern

Teat cistern: The cavity within the teat and is located just below the gland cistern. It is continuous with the gland cistern. It is lined with numerous longitudinal and circular mucosal folds, which from pocket on the inner lining of the teat.

4. What is structure of the mammary gland?

Ans. It consists of **connective tissue, ductular system** and **secretory tissue**

Connective tissue (stroma)

The function of the connective tissue is to support the ductular and the secretory tissues. A desirable udder should contain a minimal amount of connective tissue and maximal amounts of secretory tissue.

Ductular System

The ductular system of the mammary gland starts at the alveoli and ends at the streak canal. Milk is first collected in the lumen of the alveoli and secretory ductules. It then drains into larger ducts until it enters the primary (mammary) ducts attached to the **gland cistern**. The gland cistern is the largest collecting point of milk. The gland cistern is linked to the **teat cistern**. The two cisterns are partially separated by an **annular fold**. Usually 10-12 ducts lead into each gland cistern but as many as 20 ducts can be found. Milk in the teat cistern is prevented from escaping to the outside by a sphincter muscle which contracts around the **teat (streak) canal** through which milk is drawn to the outside.

Secretory Tissue

The secretory epithelial cells comprise about 1/2 of the total cells in the secretory tissue during lactation. Secretory tissue is arranged into **lobes** with each lobes consists of many **lobules**. Each lobule containing clusters or groups of **alveoli** (150-220 alveoli) which are surrounded by a network of blood vessels. Each alveolus has all the components required to produce and deliver milk to the duct system. Each alveolus consists of a single layer of **epithelial cells (secretory cells)** surrounding the **central lumen** into which the epithelial cells eject the milk they synthesize.

5. What is the precursors of Milk?

Ans. Precursors of milk come from the bloodstream. Normally 400-500 ml blood is supplied to mammary gland to synthesize one ml of milk. The primary substrates extracted from blood by the secretory cell include glucose, amino acids, fatty acids and minerals. For ruminants acetate and β- hydroxybutyrate are also major substrates extracted from the blood. Glucose is the precursor for lactose, citric acid and most of the glycerol portion of the triacylglycerol. The major carbohydrate found in the milk is lactose and only glucose is found in the blood. Several materials in milk come unchanged from the blood, including minerals, hormones and several proteins especially immunoglobulins.

6. What is milk Ejection?

Ans. **Ejection** of milk is accomplished by contraction of the myoepithelial cells surrounding each alveolus. The ejection process results in a rapid transfer of milk from the lobulo-alveolar spaces into larger ducts. The flow of milk due to passive withdrawal, which is greatly increased following ejection, is commonly known as **letdown**. In some occasions, the intramammary pressure is sufficiently great to overcome the resistance of the teat sphincter so that the milk may leak from the teat. Milk ejection is a neurohormonal reflex associated with the release of **oxytocin**. Milk ejection reflex has a neural (afferent) and a hormonal (efferent) component.

7. What are compositions of milk?

Ans. **Milk** the normal secretion of mammary gland is an emulsion of fat in a watery solution of sugar and minerals and with protein in a colloidal suspension. The principal constituents of milk are water and total solids. Total solids are mainly classified as fat (lipid) and solid not fat (SNF). Water acts as medium in which these two constituents are carried. Water is constituted around 87% of milk and total solids are around 13%. All the major constituents are synthesized in the udder from various precursors which are absorbed selectively from blood.

Water: Water is the main constituent of milk and is secreted in association with water soluble constituents like lactose, sodium, potassium and choline.

Milk fat: Milk fat is mixture of triglycerol containing mostly of saturated and partly of unsaturated fatty acids and is derived from fatty acids of the blood triglycerides or synthesized from acetate or β-hydroxy butyrate of blood plasma.

Milk sugar: Lactose is the major carbohydrate of milk. It is disaccharide composed of one molecule of glucose and one molecule of galactose. Both glucose and galactose are joined together by β1-4 glycosidic linkage. This lactose is synthesized within epithelial cells of alveoli. For lactose synthesis glucose of blood is utilized by the alveolar cells to produce galactose for ultimate production of lactose.

Milk proteins: The primary group of milk proteins are casein which are derived primarily from the amino acids of blood. There are three or four caseins in milk of most species. All other proteins found in milk are grouped together as **whey proteins**. The major whey proteins in the cow milk are **lactoglobulin** and **lactalbumin**. These milk proteins are synthesized in the mammary epithelial cells and are only produced by mammary gland. The immunoglobulins are serum albumin in milk and are not synthesized by the epithelial cells. **Caseins** have an appropriate amino acid composition that is important for growth and development of nursing young.

Ash in milk: The ash in milk are calcium, phosphorous, magnesium, potassium, chlorine, iron, manganese and iodine. There are considerable amount of vitamins like vitamin A and vitamin B and smaller quantities of vitamin C, D, E and K are found in milk. These vitamins are not synthesized in udder but are absorbed from blood like all mineral elements.

8. What is milk ejection reflex?

Ans. **Milk ejection reflex** has a neural (afferent) and a hormonal (efferent) component. Ejection of milk is accomplished by contraction of the myoepithelial cells surrounding each alveolus. The ejection process results in a rapid transfer of milk from the lobulo-alveolar spaces into larger ducts. The flow of milk due to passive withdrawal, which is greatly increased following ejection, is commonly known as **letdown**. **Milk ejection** is a neurohormonal reflex associated with the release of **oxytocin**. Oxytocin is released into the blood in response to action potential of nerve impulses originated in the teat. It then travels to the mammary gland and binds to protein receptor sites on the epithelial secretory cells. This results in contraction of the secretory cells and expulsion of milk from the mammary gland. Milk ejection can be stimulated by suckling and milking, washing the udder, presence of the young. The timing of oxytocin release relative to milk removal is an important factor affecting milk ejection. An essential component of the **milk ejection reflex** is the binding of oxytocin, specifically and with high affinity, to protein receptor sites on the **myoepithelial cells**. This results in contraction of the myoepithelial cells and expulsion of milk from the mammary gland.

9. What is colostrums and how it is different from milk?

Ans. The first secretion of mammary gland following parturition is known as **colostrum.** Colostrum contains a large proportion of albumin, globulin and minerals. Colostrum is richer in most nutrients including vitamins than milk apart from lactose and fat. The capacity of newborn to absorb antibodies from gut declines rapidly and lasts from 12-24 hrs after birth. Since placental transfer of antibodies to foetal tissues does not occur in ruminants, their neonates depends on colostrums as a source of antibodies. This passive immunity is necessary for the young until they develop active immunity.

10. How biosynthesis of milk components occurs?

Ans. Milk synthesis takes place inside epithelial cells lining the alveoli. Some milk components like vitamins, minerals and some proteins are not synthesized in the epithelial cells but are rather filtered from blood through the epithelial cells and forms components of milk. Other components like lactose, fat and most milk proteins are synthesized inside epithelial cells from various blood precursors. All filtered components and precursors of blood pass into the alveolar cells through the plasma membrane. Some blood components pass through membrane easily while others are excluded thus the plasma membrane is often called as selective semipermeable membrane.

11. How milk protein is synthesized?

Ans. The total protein components of milk is composed of numerous specific proteins. The primary group of milk proteins are casein, lactalbumin and lactglobulin are not present in blood but they are synthesized from blood precursors amino acids. These three proteins constitute about 90-95% of total protein nitrogen in cow's milk. The immunoglobulins and serum albumin appears to be identical in blood and milk and are thus diffuses in milk in unchanged form from blood. The mechanism of protein synthesis in mammary gland appears to be comparable to those found in most other protein synthesizing cells. Amino acids of blood are absorbed through the basal membrane of the epithelial cells of the mammary gland by several specific amino acid transport system. Then amino acids are covalently bound together with ribosomes on rough endoplasmic reticulum and synthesize proteins in same pattern as all proteins are synthesized in rough endoplasmic reticulum. The steps of protein synthesis include transcription, stability of m RNA and translation of mRNA to protein. After synthesis of protein these newly synthesized proteins are transferred from rough endoplasmic reticulum to golgi apparatus for post translational modification, such as chain folding, phosphorylation etc.

12. How milk glucose (lactose) is synthesized?

Ans. Lactose a disaccharide composed of glucose and galactose is the prominent carbohydrate found exclusively in milk. Lactose is the least variable component of milk and is the major and easily digestible source of glucose which provides energy to neonates. For synthesis of one molecule of lactose, two molecules of glucose must enter the mammary epithelial cells. One glucose is converted to galactose. Glucose is combined with galactose to form lactose by the enzyme lactose synthase in golgi apparatus. The detail mechanism by which lactose is synthesized is that one glucose is converted to uridine diphosphate (UDP) glucose. UDP glucose is converted to UDP galactose. Finally produced UDP galactose combines to another glucose and produce lactose in presence lactose synthase.

Glucose + ATP Hexokinase Glucose 6 Phosphate + ADP

Glucose 6 Phosphate Phosphoglucomutase Glucose 1 phosphate

Glucose 1 phosphate UDP glucose pyrophosphate UDP glucose + Pyrophosphate

UDP glucose UDP galactose 4 epimerase UDP galactose

UDP galactose + glucose Lactose synthase Lactose + UDP

12. How milk fat is synthesized?

Ans. Milk fats are characterized as a mixture of triglycerides with fatty acids (C4-C16). The fatty acid, glycerol and other related intermediates are synthesized in the cytosol and biosynthesis of triglycerides takes place in or near endoplasmic reticulum of the mammary epithelial cells. Milk fat is the most variable component of milk. There are three major source of fatty acids. The first and one of the prime importance in ruminants is synthesis of fatty acids in mammary gland from acetate and β-OH butyrate transported from rumen. Acetate in malonyl CoA pathway contributes to all short chains (C4-C14) fatty acids and to a portion of C16 fatty acid in ruminants. Ruminants can not use acetyl CoA derived from glucose for fatty acid synthesis but glucose is a major source of acetyl CoA for fatty acid synthesis in non ruminants. The second source of fatty acid is triglycerides present in circulating chylomicrons and low density lipoproteins. These fatty acids more than 14 carbons in length are of either dietary or rumen microbial origin and are mainly palmitic (C16) and stearic, oleic and linoleic (C18) acids. More than half of the fatty acids in cow's milk are derived directly from the blood, 1/3rd of these are C16 acids and most are C18 acids. The third source of fatty acid is cytoplasmic acetyl CoA from glucose through glycolysis and citric acid cycle. The primary source of triglyceride in most of the species is glycerol-3 phosphate which are derived either from glycolytic pathway or from the lipolysis of triglycerides during fatty acid uptake by mammary gland. These are two major pathways for **synthesis of triglycerides**. They are

i) ∝-glycerol phosphate pathway in which phosphatidic acids are formed. On removal of the phosphate molecule from phosphatidic acid a third long chain acyl CoA molecule is attached 1,2 diglyceride to form triglyceride.

ii) Monoglyceride pathway, which involves the formation of 1,2 diglyceride from acylation of two monoglycerides.

13. What is mammogenesis?

Ans. Mammogenesis is the term use to describe the development of the mammary gland. Mammary development begins when the animal is an early fetus and proceeds beyond initiation of lactation. The mammary gland is one of a few tissues in mammals that can repeatedly undergo growth, functional differentiation and regression.

Stages of Development in Embryo: The early embryo has three layers, which ultimately give rise to various tissues and organs of the body. These layers are ectoderm (outer layer), mesoderm (middle layer) and endoderm (inner layer). The mammary gland is derived from the ectoderm and the mesoderm layers. The **first sign** in the development of the mammary gland is the thickening of the ectodermal cells (embryonic skin) of the ventral surface of the embryo giving rise to the mammary band. In bovine, this occurs about 35 days after conception. Serial changes in the thickened area of the ectoderm are identified as the mammary band, mammary streak, mammary line, mammary crest, mammary hillock and mammary bud. Upon cell multiplication, aggregation and differentiation, four structure called **mammary buds** are formed. The mammary bud is represented by the end of the teat in the area of the streak canal. The bud is the main structure from which all mammary glands arise.

14. What is lactogenesis?

Ans. Initiation of milk secretion is called as **Lactogenesis.** It is a series of cellular changes whereby mammary epithelial cells are converted from a non secretory state to a secretory state. This process is normally associated with the end of pregnancy and around the time of parturition. Lactogenesis is a two stage process. Biochemical changes occur in the mammary gland as it turns from inactive to an active stage. There is a marked increase in the RNA level of the epithelial cells.

15. What is galactopoeisis?

Ans. Galactopoeisis is defined as the maintenance of lactation or milk secretion once lactation has been established. The changes in mammary cell numbers (by growth or cell death) and in milk yield per cell are regulated by galactopoietic hormones and local mammary factors. Without frequent emptying of the mammary gland milk synthesis will not persist in spite of adequate hormonal status. Conversely, maintenance of intense suckling or milking stimulus will not maintain lactation indefinitely. Nevertheless, suckling or actual removal of milk is required to maintain lactation.

16. What is the role of hormones on galactopoieisis?

Ans. The maintenance of lactation is controlled by a group of hormones collectively known as galactopoeitic hormonal complex. The hormonal complex includes prolactin, growth hormones, thyroid hormones and glucocorticoids.

Prolactin: In most nonruminants and ruminants prolactin is only one component of a hormonal complex that regulates galactopoeisis. The role prolactin in cows is ambiguous. There is milking-induced or nursing-induced release of prolactin. The milking-induced prolactin surge is a direct link between the act of nursing and the galactopoeitic hormones involved in maintaining lactation.

Growth hormone: Growth hormone is essential for maintaining lactation (galactopoeitic). Growth hormone coordinates changes in body tissues and physiological processes that support increase in synthesis of lactose, protein and fat in the mammary gland. Bovine somatotropin or bovine growth hormone is now commercially produced and has been used in many dairy herds to increase milk yield. An increase in milk yield of 10 40% has been reported. The use of BST is not permitted in India and Canada.

Adrenal Corticoids: Intact adrenal gland is essential for maintaining lactation. Glucocorticoids at physiological levels is galactopoeitic, however, at high doses it inhibits lactation.

Thyroid Hormones: Thyroid hormones are galactopoeitic. Injection of thyroid hormone into cows increases milk production for a short period of time. Administration of thyroid hormones for more that 7 weeks had no effect on milk yield. There are generally no benefit in feeding thyroprotein over the entire lactation.

Ovarian Hormones: Estrogen administered in very low doses is galactopoietic. However, higher doses have inhibitory effects. A combination of estrogen and progesterone is more inhibitory than estrogen alone. Progesterone alone has no effect on galactopoeisis because there are no progesterone receptors in the mammary gland during lactation

17. What is mammary gland involution?

Ans. After peak yield of milk which occurs within few days or weak after parturition in most species there is decrease in milk secretion takes place. This decrease in milk secretion is primarily due to involution of mammary gland tissue. Mammary gland involution takes place after the peak lactation and after cessation of milking process or suckling of young. The cessation of milk removal has a more drastic effect on the involution process than that due to natural involution after peak lactation. Involution is due to a combination of decrease in cell numbers and the secretion rate of mammary cells.

18. What is mastitis?

Ans. Mastitis is an inflammatory reaction of the mammary gland to bacterial, chemical, thermal or mechanical injury. This inflammation may be characterized by gross swelling, heat, readness, pain and disturbed function of mammary gland that finally results in decrease in milk production and change in milk composition. The most common mastitis causing pathogens are staphylococci and streptococci. Yeast like candida albicans may also cause mastitis. The main route of entry of causative agent for mastitis are through teat canal. Depending on severity and onset of symptoms mastitis are classified into peracute, acute, subacute and chronic mastitis. Test to detect mastitis is to measure the concentration of lecucocytes in milk by **stripcup** and **california mastitis test**.

Choose the Best Answer

1. Rennin is required for digestion of

a) Albumin b) Caesin
c) Globulin d) Fibrinoge

2. Milk sugar is

a) Lactose b) Glucose
c) Fructose d) Galactose

3. Average lactation period of cow is

a) 105 days b) 205 days
c) 305 days d) 405 days

4. Infection in udder cause

a) Metritis b) Mastitis
c) Colitis d) Stenosis

5. Milk production is not

a) Season dependent b) Discontineous process
c) Weather dependent d) Contineous process

6. Mammary glands are

a) Modified sebaceous gland b) Modified salivary gland
c) Modifies sweat gland d) Endocrine gland

7. Milk is ________ to blood

a) Isotonic b) Hypotonic
c) Hypertonic d) Variable

8. Hormone responsible for milk ejection is

a) Thyroxine b) Adrenal
c) Estrogen d) Oxytocin

9. Milk fever is characterized by

a) Decrease in Ca^{+2} in plasma b) Increase in Ca^{+2} in plasma
c) Decrease in Na^{+} in plasma d) Increase in Na^{+} in plasma

10. Which constituent is less in colostrums

a) Lactose b) Antibody
c) Carotene d) Lipids

11. Hormone responsible for milk formation is

a) GH b) Prolactin
c) Aldosterone d) Calcitonin

12. Hypomagnesium in calf causes

a) Milk fever b) Bloat
c) Grass tetany d) Acidosis

13. Let down of milk is stimulated by

a) Low temperature b) Sight of calf
c) Voice of calf d) Suckling of calves

14. Excess secretion of which hormone causes "holding up" the milk

a) Oxytocin b) Adrenalin
c) Estrogen d) Prolactin

15. Plasma protein which is abundantly found in colostrums is

a) Globulin b) Albumin
c) Angiotensin d) Fibrinogen

16. Mammary gland is originate from

a) Endoderm b) Ectoderm
c) Mesoderm d) Both a & c

17. Milk is

a) Slightly acidic (pH 6.8) b) Slightly basic (pH 7.4)
c) Neutral d) Highly basic

18. Ideal dry period of cow is

a) 8 weeks b) 3 weeks
c) 11 weeks d) 10 weeks

19. Quantity of milk production does not depend on

a) Age b) Breed
c) Feed d) Coat colour

20. Number of teats in goat is

a) 1 b) 2
c) 3 d) 4

21. Milking twice daily yields _______ milk than milking once daily

a) More b) Less
c) Equal d) Double

22. Functional unit of lactating mammary gland is

a) Alveolus b) Lobe
c) Lobule d) Gland cistern

23. Colostrum gives passive immunity by

a) Vit A/Carotene b) Globulin
c) Casein d) Lactose

24. Initiation of milk secretion is termed as

a) Mammogenesis b) Lactogenesis
c) Galactogenesis d) Lactation

25. In ruminants placental transfer of antibodies

a) Takes Place
b) Doesn't occur
c) Occurs but in small amount
d) Occurs only after partuirition

26. As day advances amount of carotene in milk of lactating cow

a) Increases b) Decreases
c) Remains equal d) Can'tbe predicted

27. Mammary lobes consists of

a) Teat cistern b) Lobules
c) Streak canal d) Gland cistern

28. Milk comes out of udder through

a) Alveolus b) Lobes
c) Teat cistern d) Streak canal

29. Two halves of bovine udder is separated by

a) Lateral suspensory ligament
b) Median suspensory ligament
c) Horizontal suspensory ligament
d) Vertical suspensory ligament

30. Mammary gland are _____ in nature

a) Holocrine b) Epi/Merocrine
c) Apocrine d) Both a & b

31. Ketone bodies are found in milk in case of

a) Ketosis b) Acidosis
c) Bloat d) Milk fever

32. Mammary glands are

a) Compound tubular b) Compound alveolar
c) Simple tubular d) Compound tubuloalveoplar

33. Let down of milk stops after 10-20min of milking because of

a) Fatigue of myoepithelial cells
b) Sympathetic nervous system
c) Inactivation of Oxytocin
d) Activation of Prolactin

34. Milk synthesizing epithelial cells are present in

a) Gland cistern
b) Streak canal
c) Alveoli
d) Teat cistern

35. Mammogenesis is

a) Milk production
b) Growth and development of mammary gland
c) Muscle contraction
d) Udder infection

36. Milk fever can be treated by

a) Oral administration of Vit. D
b) Drying of the cows
c) Injection of Oxytocin
d) Feeding more water

37. The process of differentiation where by the mammary alveolar cells acquire the ability to secrete milk is called as

a) Mammogenesis
b) Lactogenesis
c) Induction of milk synthesis
d) Both b & c

38. Lactation is absent in

a) Cow
b) Whale
c) Cat
d) Fowl

39. Organ mainly involved in glucose metabolism during lactation is

a) Mammary gland
b) Liver
c) Pancrease
d) Kidney

40. Metabolic adaptation are associated with onset of lactation in glucose metabolism

a) Increased gluconeogenesis and Increased glucogenolysis
b) Decreased gluconeogenesis and Increased glucogenolysis
c) Decreased gluconeogenesis and Decreased glucogenolysis
d) Increased gluconeogenesis and Decreased glucogenolysis

41. With the onset of lactation the utilization of acetate for energy in glucose metabolism occurs in which tissue/organ of ruminants

a) Adipose tissue b) Mammary gland
c) Liver d) Muscles

42. During lactation changes occurs in lipid metabolism are

a) Increase in Lipolysis and decrease in lipogenesis
b) Decrease in Lipolysis and increase in lipogenesis
c) Increase in Lipolysis and Increase in lipogenesis
d) Decrease in Lipolysis and decrease in lipogenesis

43. The predominant immunoglobulin in bovine colostrums is

a) IgA b) IgE
c) IgG d) IgM

44. Lactose is a disaccharide composed of

a) Glucose and Fructose b) Glucose and Galactose
c) Galactose and Fructose d) Fructose and Mannose

45. Milk protein is synthesize in which part of cell

a) Golgi complex b) Rough ER
c) Smooth ER d) Mitochondria

46. Milk that is left in the mammary gland after complete normal milking or suckling is called as

a) Calf milk b) Temporary milk
c) Residual milk d) Permanent milk

47. Percentage of residual milk may range from

a) 0-10% b) 5-10%
c) 10-20% d) 20-30%

48. In the milk fat the carbon chain of fatty acids ranges from

a) C1-C5
b) C4-C16
c) C17-C22
d) C23-C30

49. Ideal dry period for cow is

a) 2-5wk
b) 6-8wk
c) 3months
d) 4months

50. Milking twice daily yield at least ________% more milk than milking once daily

a) 10%
b) 20%
c) 30%
d) 40%

51. Milking thrice daily yield at least ________% more milk than milking twice daily

a) 0-5%
b) 5-20%
c) 15-30%
d) 20-40%

52. The milk removal/milk ejection is a

a) Hormonal control
b) Neural control
c) Both a & b
d) Physical process

53. Hormone which is not associated with lactogenesis is

a) Progesterone
b) Testosterone
c) Prolactin
d) Insulin

54. Marked increase in milk yield after parturition in cows reaches to maximum yield at

a) 1st week
b) 2-8 week
c) 8-14 week
d) 14-20 week

55. Overall daily capacity for energy transfer via milk is rather constant in mammary species

a) 100 kcal/kg 0.75 body weight
b) 125 kcal/kg 0.75 body weight
c) 150 kcal/kg 0.75 body weight
d) 175 kcal/kg 0.75 body weight

56. Thermo neutral zone where the milk yield is nearly constant

a) 5-10°C b) 10-20°C
c) 20-30°C d) 30-35°C

57. At the time of milk ejection the intra-mammary pressure increases upto

a) 10-20 mmHg b) 20-35 mmHg
c) 35-55 mmHg d) 55-75 mmHg

58. Physiological factors that contribute to increase production with frequent milking are

a) Less intra-mammary pressure
b) Increased stimulation by hormone
c) Less negative feed back on the cellular synthesis as a result of build up of milk components
d) All of the above

Answers

1. b	2. a	3. c	4. b	5. b	6. c	7. a	8. d	9. a	10. a
11. b	12. c	13. d	14. b	15. a	16. b	17. a	18. a	19. d	20. b
21. a	22. a	23. b	24. b	25. b	26. b	27. b	28. d	29. b	30. c
31. a	32. d	33. c	34. c	35. b	36. a	37. d	38. d	39. b	40. a
41. b	42. a	43. c	44. b	45. b	46. c	47. c	48. b	49. b	50. d
51. b	52. c	53. b	54. b	55. b	56. b	57. c	58. d		

□□□

CHAPTER-13

Behavioral Physiology

1. What is behavior?

Ans. Study of animal behavior is called **ethology**. **Behavior** is the expressed sum of individual muscle contractions and hormonal secretion. Behavior is the result of the way the various nervous systems interact with each other and with the internal and external world. Concept of behavior alters an animal's relationship to its external world. One of the principal consequences of behavior is adjustment of the sensory input.

2. What is ingestive behavior or feeding behavior?

Ans. This type of behavior is an important sign of health as it is means of converting plants into meat or hair. Various species chew their food in different ways. Rabbit and other rodents nibble their feed with sharp incisors. Horse grasp forage with heir teeth where as cattle use tongue for this. Sheep graze much close to the ground than cattle because of the flexibility of their cleft upper lip. Special feeding pattern characterize certain species like pigs while feeding root and turn over the soil, rabbit is known for its coprophagus nature and dogs bury bones and carry food from one place to another. Social influence also affect feeding. It is observed that group fed animals tend to eat more. The patterns of ingestive behavior are related to the anatomy and physiology of each species and the nature of its characteristic food. Because of its economic importance this behavior has been studied detail in many species.

3. What is grazing behavior?

Ans. Cattle and sheep graze mostly in day light beginning around sun rise and ending about sun dawn. If day temperature is high cattle will graze more at night. Cattle generally function as social unit in which every member engaging in grazing, exploring and ruminating at the same time. Goats are browsers because they have no taste receptors so they enjoy a wide variety of plants that are distasteful to other species. Grazing distance varies with climate, topography, availability of forage and species. On an average catle graze about 3miles/ day. Sheep travels about 3-8 miles/day.

4. What is pheromones?

Ans. Pheromone commonly modulate sexual behavior. Ex. Attraction of male dogs to bitch in estrus. In rodents male sex pheromones in urine can accelerate the onset of puberty in young female. Pheromones sometimes regulate maternal behavior as mother sometimes reject reject heir newborn because they smell wrong. Similar rejection can occur if a new mother is given new born from another mother or even if its own new born becomes contaminated with odors from human handling.

□□□